Diagnosis and Management of Multiple Sclerosis

WITHDRAWN

First Edition

John O. Fleming, MD

Professor and Vice-Chairman
Department of Neurology
Professor, Department of Medical
Microbiology and Immunology
Director of the Multiple Sclerosis Clinic
University of Wisconsin–Madison Medical School

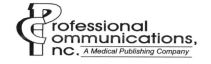

Professional Communications, Inc.
A Medical Publishing Company

Published by
Professional Communications, Inc.

Marketing Office:
400 Center Bay Drive
West Islip, NY 11795
(t) 631/661-2852
(f) 631/661-2167

Editorial Office:
PO Box 10
Caddo, OK 74729-0010
(t) 580/367-9838
(f) 580/367-9989

ISBN: 1-884735-32-0

Printed in the United States of America

For orders only, please call:
1-800-337-9838
Or visit our website:
www.pcibooks.com

DISCLAIMER
The opinions expressed in this publication reflect those of the author. However, the author makes no warranty regarding the contents of the publication. The protocols described herein are general and may not apply to a specific patient. Any product mentioned in this publication should be taken in accordance with the prescribing information provided by the manufacturer.

This text is printed on recycled paper.

DEDICATION

To my wife, Barbara, and children, Michael and Kristin, whose sacrifices have made this work possible; Dr. Kolar Murthy, truly a clinician's clinician and my first teacher in neurology; Dr. Leslie Weiner, my mentor, whose maxim was "to bring the clinic to the laboratory and the laboratory to the clinic," and, finally, my courageous patients, who have taught me so much about this disease, who have been understanding when I have been wrong, and whose patience has far exceeded anything their doctor could reasonably expect.

ACKNOWLEDGMENT

I wish to thank the following colleagues for generously reviewing parts of the manuscript and providing helpful suggestions and criticisms: Brad Beinlich, John Christianson, Donald Goodkin, Victor Haughton, Norman Kachuck, Lorri Lobeck, Sheila McKee , Lisa Okon-Lowndes, Loren Rolak, Howard Rowley, and Raymond Sobel. Nevertheless, all errors that remain are entirely my own.

The author also gratefully acknowledges Gina Chijimatsu, Nikki D. Weaver, and Phyllis Jones Freeny for excellent assistance with manuscript preparation and editorial revision.

About the Author

Dr. Fleming graduated from Colgate University (BA) and the State University of New York in Brooklyn (MD). He completed residencies in internal medicine at UCLA–Wadsworth and neurology at Cornell–Northshore, and he is board-certified in both of these specialties. He undertook additional neurological training at the National Hospital, Queen Square, London; Maida Vale Hospital (under Professor Ian McDonald), London; UCLA–Wadsworth (multiple sclerosis fellowship under Dr. Wallace Tourtellotte); and USC (neurovirology fellowship under Dr. Leslie Weiner and Dr. Stephen Stohlman). He has pursued laboratory research with animal models of multiple sclerosis, and he has been a participant or principal investigator in clinical trials of disease-modifying treatments for multiple sclerosis.

He has been a recipient of research grant support from the National Institutes of Health and the National Multiple Sclerosis Society and has served as a member of scientific study section advisory committees for both of these institutions. In the Department of Neurology at the University of Wisconsin, Madison, he has served as Director of the Multiple Sclerosis Clinic, Director of the Residency Program, Acting Chair, and Vice Chair. He also is a faculty member in the Virology Program and the Department of Medical Microbiology and Immunology at the University of Wisconsin. He has no commercial or financial relationships to disclose.

TABLE OF CONTENTS

TABLES

FIGURES

Introduction

Multiple sclerosis (MS) is a common neurological disorder and an important cause of disability in young adults. For example, in the United States, 350,000 individuals are afflicted with this disease. Physicians in every field of medicine will encounter patients with MS, and thus there is a need for all clinicians to be familiar with this disease and comfortable with its management, whether this be in the role of specialist or general practitioner.

The purpose of this handbook is to provide a summary of MS diagnosis and treatment from the perspective of the busy clinician who must evaluate, treat, and follow-up patients with different manifestations of this disease. The primary emphasis has been on practical first-line management strategies which are usually effective and benefit the majority of patients; additionally, suggestions for management or referral of complex or refractory cases are provided.

Long regarded as an enigmatic, untreatable, and crippling degenerative condition, MS is starting to yield its secrets to the advances of modern biomedical research. An understanding of disease mechanisms is emerging and several effective disease-modifying treatments have been identified. These findings have been summarized and the primary literature cited in the present handbook. Nevertheless, in a short text, it is impossible to adequately acknowledge the advances made by the numerous scientists and clinicians who have studied MS. For a more complete discussion, additional printed and electronic resources are noted in the final chapter; in particular, the indicated reference texts comprehensively review all scientific and clinical aspects of MS and are highly recommended.

It is not surprising that the dramatic explosion in scientific understanding of MS is associated with unresolved questions and even controversy. For example, currently, there is vigorous debate with regard to the long-term benefits of early treatment in MS and mono-symptomatic demyelination. I have cited authorities either strongly favoring or seriously questioning early treatment. Nevertheless, it is instructive that a careful reading of statements from participants on both sides of this debate indicates agreement that in the absence of rigorous long-term studies, the value of treatment over decades, the relevant time frame for this chronic neurological disease, is *unknown*. By definition, without long-term studies, long-term effects are not known.

With regard to the advisability of early treatment and other controversial issues in MS management I have attempted to present a middle-of-the-road, evidence-based approach consistent with the current practice of most experienced neurologists in North America. Given the imperfect state of our present knowledge and the likelihood that future research will alter treatment guidelines, the strategy I have recommended is based on common sense, a healthy skepticism of dogmatic statements, an individualized approach to patient management, and full, informed consent. In an active practice with diverse patients, I have found it especially helpful to involve patients in treatment decisions, indicating what is and is not known, and giving strong weight to each patient's perception of the acceptability of different courses of action. In this regard, the statement of Dr. Labe Scheinberg several years ago concerning therapeutic strategies in MS is relevant:

> *Some of the things I will mention are so basic to the tenets of medical practice that I am embarrassed to mention them here, except that from my observations, they are so often neglected in the daily management of MS patients that they need restatement.*[334]

The management of MS may be challenging, and the deficits which patients develop are at times heart-breaking. On the other hand, the care of patients with MS is usually very satisfying, as we are emerging from an era of therapeutic nihilism, and patients are extremely appreciative for the diagnostic and therapeutic measures that their physicians provide and that help them to better cope with this cruel disease. It is my hope that this handbook will be of practical benefit to practitioners in this endeavor.

1   Definition and Pathology

Introduction

Multiple sclerosis (MS) typically commences with episodic, relapsing-remitting neurological symptoms in a young adult. Common presentations include:

- Monocular visual disturbances due to optic neuritis
- Paresthesias or weakness caused by spinal cord involvement
- Incoordination provoked by lesions in the cerebellum
- Diplopia as a result of brain stem dysfunction.

At autopsy, MS is characterized by multiple discrete areas of myelin loss and gliosis throughout the white matter of brain and spinal cord—the classic plaques of demyelination (Figure 1.1). Thus the hallmark of MS is a neurological disease pattern that is disseminated in space (multiple central nervous system [CNS] lesions) and time (recurrent attacks). The "gold standard" for diagnosis is the disease course above, coupled with characteristic plaques on pathological examination. Magnetic resonance imaging (MRI) is approaching the ideal of revealing macroscopic pathology in the living patient and therefore has led to a revolution in the diagnosis and study of MS. Nonetheless, MRI appearances often are nonspecific, and only pathological examination can reveal events at the microscopic level that provide clues as to the cellular mechanisms of MS.

FIGURE 1.1 — CLASSIC PATHOLOGY OF MULTIPLE SCLEROSIS

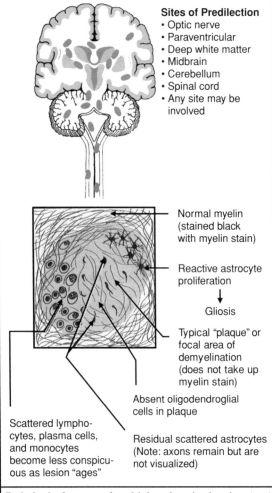

Sites of Predilection
- Optic nerve
- Paraventricular
- Deep white matter
- Midbrain
- Cerebellum
- Spinal cord
- Any site may be involved

Normal myelin (stained black with myelin stain)

Reactive astrocyte proliferation

↓

Gliosis

Typical "plaque" or focal area of demyelination (does not take up myelin stain)

Absent oligodendroglial cells in plaque

Residual scattered astrocytes (Note: axons remain but are not visualized)

Scattered lymphocytes, plasma cells, and monocytes become less conspicuous as lesion "ages"

Pathologic features of multiple sclerosis showing *(top)* the common locations at which plaques of demyelination occur and *(bottom)* the histologic features of a plaque.

Reference 63.

Clinical Subtypes of Multiple Sclerosis

As indicated, MS patients commonly have a course characterized by episodic bouts of abrupt worsening. These attacks, or relapses, usually last several weeks and typically are followed by at least partial recovery or remission. Pathological and MRI investigations have shown that relapses are associated with new lesions of CNS demyelination, the plaques shown in Figure 1.1. Patients with this episodic, recurring pattern of disease activity are classified as suffering from relapsing-remitting MS (RRMS).

Eventually, a substantial number of patients with RRMS will develop a pattern of gradual progression, though superimposed relapses may or may not continue; the disease course of such patients is designated secondary-progressive MS (SPMS). Also, a minority of patients will have a disease course that is progressive *from onset*, either without relapses (primary-progressive MS [PPMS]) or with superimposed relapses (progressive-relapsing MS [PRMS]). Several studies have indicated that the distinction between PPMS and PRMS may not be significant biologically[401]; however, the two terms are retained in this handbook because of their use in scientific reports and pharmaceutical regulations. The older term "chronic progressive MS" has largely been abandoned in favor of the more precise terms for progressive forms of disease, ie, SPMS, PPMS, and PRMS.

The four types of MS disease course are illustrated in Figure 1.2. Note that the most important distinction—between a relapsing and progressive pattern—is made on the basis of the slope of neurological disability plotted against time. Relapses are characterized by a defined, abrupt worsening of symptoms; the patient can usually name the day that a distinctly new symptom occurred. By contrast, progression is manifest by a gradual, insidious increase of disability. The

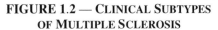

FIGURE 1.2 — CLINICAL SUBTYPES OF MULTIPLE SCLEROSIS

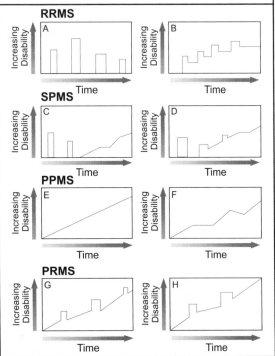

Relapsing-remitting multiple sclerosis (RRMS) is characterized by clearly defined acute attacks with full recovery (A) or with sequelae and residual deficit upon recovery (B). Periods between disease relapses are characterized by lack of disease progression. Secondary progressive MS (SPMS) begins with an initial RR course, followed by progression of variable rate (C) that may also include occasional relapses and minor remissions (D). Primary progressive MS (PPMS) is characterized by disease showing progression of disability from onset, without plateaus or remissions (E) or with occasional plateaus and temporary minor improvements (F). Progressive-relapsing MS (PRMS) shows progression from onset but with clear acute relapses with (G) or without (H) full recovery.

Reference 214.

patient notes steady worsening over the past months or years but is unable to clearly specify a date when symptoms suddenly intensified.

The relative proportions of MS patients with each disease subtype will vary with populations under study and physician referral patterns. As an example, a prevalence study of 3019 patients in New York State revealed[238]:

- RRMS—55%
- SPMS—31%
- PPMS—9%
- PRMS—5%.

The four disease types above are well-established, particularly with application to clinical trials of new medications. As a result, approved therapies usually are subtype-specific (see Chapter 6, *Disease-Modifying Treatment*). Currently, there is not a robust correlation between the four clinical subtypes defined by disease course and classifications based on pathology or MRI, although a major goal of current research is to establish better correlations.

Classic Pathology

The classic pathological features of MS are illustrated in Figure 1.1.[63] Macroscopically, the predilection of lesions for sites near the ventricular surface or in the deep white matter is evident (Figure 1.1A), although occasional involvement of cerebral cortex and deep gray matter nuclei has also been documented.[356] Microscopically, MS plaques are characterized by inflammatory infiltrates of lymphocytes, plasma cells, and monocytes; loss of myelin; relative preservation of axons; and reactive astrogliosis (Figure 1.1B). Ultrastructural studies, such as those of Prineas and Connell,[302] have demonstrated phagocytosis of myelin from morphologically intact axons (Figure 1.3), and

FIGURE 1.3 — ULTRASTRUCTURAL DEMONSTRATION OF MYELIN STRIPPING BY MACROPHAGES

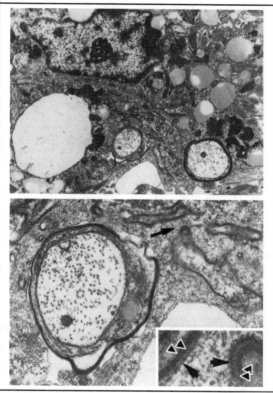

A macrophage closely invests two myelinated fibers in periplaque white matter. The sheath on the left is loose and has been partly taken up by the macrophage *(top)*. The bottom image shows this at higher magnification. The insert is an enlarged view of the area indicated by the arrow and shows myelin entering the cell in the form of two major dense lines (arrowheads) which are separated by a constant gap from the plasma membrane of the macrophage (arrows) which exhibits, on the right, the electron-dense undercoat of a coated pit.

Reference 302.

on the basis of these and other observations, it is thought that monocytic cells (macrophages/microglia) are the final effectors that cause demyelination in MS. In this regard, Sriram and Rodriguez[360] have proposed that microglial activation is the crucial event in MS pathogenesis. On the basis of these findings showing selective loss of myelin, MS has been classified as a prototypic demyelinating disease.

Recent Pathology Research

Recent studies have led to a modification, or revision, of the classical pathological description above. Two observations have been particularly pivotal in this regard:

- The demonstration of prominent axonal pathology in MS
- The delineation of heterogeneity of MS lesions, suggestive of distinct pathological subtypes.

These findings have been appreciated and well-described by neuropathologists previously[356] and even in part were made by Charcot in the 19th century. New methodology has led to an increased appreciation of the importance and implications of axonal pathology and lesion variability, as described below.

In 1997 Ferguson and colleagues[116] reported abnormal accumulation of amyloid protein in axons during MS demyelination. Subsequently, in a landmark study, Trapp and associates[383] used specific immunostaining and confocal microscopy to demonstrate axonal transection, most prominently in active, inflammatory MS lesions, as shown in Figure 1.4 and summarized in Table 1.1.[383] Importantly, axonal damage was noted in lesions that appeared early by pathological criteria, suggesting that irreversible changes begin at the onset of MS.

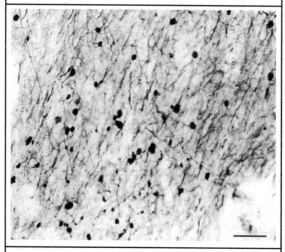

Neurofilaments in axons appear dark in this immuno-stained section of white matter from a multiple sclerosis patient. Continuous lines indicate normal, intact axons, while interrupted lines or lines terminating in ovoid swellings indicate damaged, transected axons. The scale bar represents 60 μm.

Reference 383.

Recently, Lucchinetti and colleagues[215] collected a large series of MS biopsy and autopsy specimens from three international centers. These samples were systematically studied by immunocytochemistry, using an extensive panel of monoclonal and polyclonal antibodies. As shown in Table 1.2, four distinct patterns of multiple sclerosis lesions were observed. Remarkably, analysis of the autopsy data showed that within a given patient, *only one of the four pathological subtypes of lesions was demonstrable*; in other words, the pattern of disease was completely consistent within each patient (Table 1.3). (It is important not to con-

1

TABLE 1.1 — MEAN NUMBER OF TRANSECTED AXONS IN MULTIPLE SCLEROSIS

Lesion or Area	Transected Axons/mm³
Control Patients	
Normal white matter	0.7
Multiple Sclerosis Patients	
Normal appearing nonlesion white matter	17
Chronic active lesion, center	875
Chronic active lesion, edge	3,138
Active lesions	11,236

Note the dramatic increase of transected axons in active multiple sclerosis (MS) lesions in comparison with white matter (WM) in normal control patients and normal-appearing white matter in MS patients.

Adapted from Reference 383.

fuse these proposed *pathological* subtypes defined histologically with the four well-established *clinical* subtypes of MS defined by disease course.) The homogeneity or uniformity of pathological subtype within each patient, coupled with the heterogeneity or variation of subtypes between patients, suggests that "the mechanisms and targets of demyelination in MS may be fundamentally different in distinct subgroups or stages of the disease."[215]

As Ludwin[218] points out, the recent appreciation of axonal pathology and lesion heterogeneity in MS must be confirmed by further studies, and, currently, the implications of this research should be interpreted with caution. Additionally, there is a pressing need to combine the insights of these two lines of investigation; for example, to determine if axonal damage is preferentially associated with a given pathological subtype or stage of lesion development. Correlative investigations using MRI technology may illuminate pat-

TABLE 1.2 — STRUCTURAL AND IMMUNOLOGICAL FEATURES OF DIFFERENT PATTERNS OF ACTIVE MULTIPLE SCLEROSIS LESIONS

Characteristics	Type I	Type II	Type III	Type IV
Infiltrates	T cell, Mac	T cell, Mac	T cell, Mac	T cell, Mac
Plaque geography	PV, sharp edge	PV, sharp edge	Not PV, diffuse edge	± PV, sharp edge
IgG and complement	—	++ (in areas of active demyelination)	—	—
Oligodendrocyte loss	Variable	Variable	Marked, with apoptosis	Marked, without apoptosis
Myelin protein loss	Even	Even	Predominantly MAG	Even
Clinical association (tentative)	All MS subtypes?	All MS subtypes?	Early, acute MS?	Primary progressive MS?
Possible pathogenic mechanism	Autoimmune, Mac-mediated	Autoimmune, mediated by T cells and antibody	Oligodendrogliopathy pattern similar to that observed in viral and toxic animal model diseases	Oligodendrogliopathy, unknown etiology

Abbreviations: Mac, macrophages and microglia; MAG, myelin associated glycoprotein; MS, multiple sclerosis; PV, perivenous pattern of demyelination.

The authors of this study state that the results are "a first indication" that MS may be characterized by different pathological mechanisms and that the four patterns/mechanisms indicated are suggested by analogy with other diseases and experimental models; in other words, the investigators express an appropriate degree of caution with regard to the current findings and indicate further research must be performed before the implications of the patterns above are fully understood.

Adapted from Reference 215.

TABLE 1.3 — DISTRIBUTION OF DEMYELINATING PATTERNS WITH MULTIPLE SCLEROSIS CASES (AUTOPSY DATA)

Number of Autopsy Cases (Individuals)	Total Number of Active Lesions Identified	Type I	Type II	Type III	Type IV
1	3	3/3	—	—	—
16	115	—	115/115	—	—
7	43	—	—	43/43	—
3	9	—	—	—	9/9

The distribution of lesions in 27 patients studied at autopsy is presented. Note the complete uniformity of pathological type (defined in Table 1.2 and text) within each patient. For example, in the 7 patients with type III pathology, 43 lesions were identified, *all* of which were type III; in any patient with type III lesions, no lesions of type I, II, or IV were identified.

Adapted from Reference 215.

terns of axonal loss, atrophy, lesion heterogeneity, and other informative pathological features in living patients, and substantial progress has already been made in this regard.

Despite the preceding cautions, even at this stage of our knowledge the new pathological findings raise important questions. For example, if MS is characterized by axonal pathology early in the disease course, an impetus for early anti-inflammatory treatment exists, particularly if therapy is demonstrated to influence subsequent axonal loss. Also, if MS is heterogeneous at the pathological level, ie, characterized by fundamentally different mechanisms of tissue damage in different sets of patients, in the future it may be proper to tailor treatment strategies to specific types of MS defined by presumed pathophysiology. For example, immunosupressive treatment might be administered to patients with autoimmunity, and neuroprotective medication given to patients with primary oligodendrocyte dystrophy. Clearly, further research is required to settle these important questions; nevertheless, it is realistic to hope that forthcoming answers will lead to significant advances in MS management.

For example, recently Chang and associates[417] have demonstrated that premyelinating oligodendrocytes are present in chronic MS lesions. In other words, repair of lesions with new myelin is not limited by an absence of oligodendrocyte precursors; instead, remyelination appears to be actively inhibited by a factor, possibly axonal nonreceptivity, which prevents these cells from producing myelin. If the factor inhibiting premyelinating oligodendrocyte function could be identified and counteracted, it might be possible to repair MS lesions and restore function.

2 Epidemiology and Genetics

Epidemiology

Epidemiological studies have demonstrated several major, consistent findings concerning the occurrence of multiple sclerosis (MS)[73,102,103,262,326]:

- *Latitude effect*. MS prevalence increases with increasing distance from the equator in both northern and southern hemispheres (Figure 2.1). At high latitudes, MS affects approximately 0.1% of the population (Figure 2.2).

- *Sex susceptibility*. MS is more common (approximately 2:1) in women; also, statistically, the level of MS activity lessens during pregnancy and increases in the postpartum period.

- *Migration effect*. Study of migrants to and from areas with different MS prevalences suggests that subsequent risk of developing MS is influenced by location in childhood (10 to 15 years of age). For example, residence in a relatively high-risk northern area such as the United Kingdom during adolescence is associated with a high-risk of MS development, even during subsequent migration to a relatively low-risk area such as the West Indies.

- *Epidemics*. Several outbreaks of MS have been described; also, some studies of well-defined geographic populations suggest that the incidence of MS may be increasing significantly. On the other hand, clustering may be due to chance, and increases in measured MS inci-

FIGURE 2.1 — LATITUDE EFFECT: WORLDWIDE PREVALENCE OF MULTIPLE SCLEROSIS

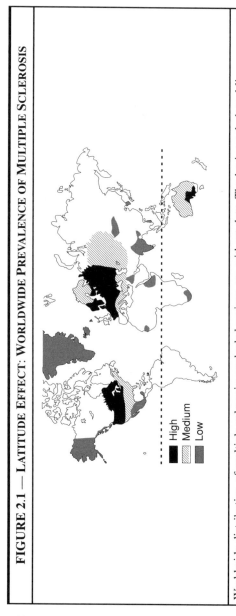

High
Medium
Low

Worldwide distribution of multiple sclerosis: unshaded regions are without data. The horizontal, dotted line represents the equator. (Prevalence risk defined as: high, at least 30 to 80 multiple sclerosis (MS) patients per 10^5 population; medium, 5 to 25/10^5; and low, <5/10^5.)

Reference 206.

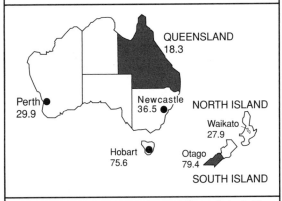

FIGURE 2.2 — LATITUDE EFFECT: RISK OF MULTIPLE SCLEROSIS IN AUSTRALIA AND NEW ZEALAND

Prevalence of multiple sclerosis (per 10^5 population). Note that even in the relatively homogenous white population of Australia and New Zealand, most of whom have ancestors from the British Isles, there is a greater than four-fold increase in multiple sclerosis risk as latitude increases.

Reference 103.

dence may be due in part to better ascertainment and diagnosis.

- *Infectious associations.* The high prevalence of MS in temperate zones is similar to the distribution of several microbes, such as viruses; additionally, evidence from serological and isolation studies has indicated a putative link between MS and different microbes. MS risk also seems increased in individuals who are exposed to common childhood infections at an older age, relative to the general population. Despite these associations and intensive, ongoing research, currently no definite association of MS with a given microbe has been confirmed.

- *Disease associations.* There is evidence that MS may be linked to other conditions such as uveitis, thyroid disease, and autoimmune conditions, thought in part to be triggered by environmental agents such as microbes.

The preceding evidence suggests that environmental determinants may be of crucial importance to MS etiology and pathogenesis. Migration studies are particularly compelling: if one can change one's risk of MS by changing one's location, then clearly, some factor in the environment is relevant. Similarly, if a given genetically defined population experiences a sudden epidemic or increase of disease, it would seem that a new environmental exposure is at work.

Unfortunately, all of the preceding epidemiological evidence is subject to potential confounders, methodological controversies, and questions of interpretation.[262] An additional problem is that the putative environmental trigger or factor(s) linked to MS has never been conclusively identified, preventing mechanistic studies focusing on one agent, such as a key virus or toxic exposure. Even more significantly, there have been countervailing studies that strongly argue for the primacy of genetic, rather than environmental, influences in determining MS risk.

Genetics

Research has also consistently identified genetic associations in MS[74,266]:
- *MS risk increases with increasing genetic relatedness.* Thus the prevalence of MS is about 1/1000 in high-risk Caucasian populations in Northern Europe or North America, and it rises to about one third in identical twins (Table 2.1). Note that in "controlled" comparisons in which shared environment is constant but the degree

of genetic relatedness varies, increased risk consistently correlates with genetic relatedness (adopted versus biological children; siblings versus half-siblings; dizygotic [DZ] [fraternal] versus monozygotic [MZ] [identical] twins).

2

- *Familial aggregations.* Approximately 10% to 15% of MS index cases have an affected relative with multiple sclerosis. However, even in extended multigenerational pedigrees with several affected individuals (multiplex families), inheritance does not follow a simple mendelian pattern, indicating that the genetics of MS is complex. The rate of conjugal MS, that is, the occurrence of MS in the exposed spouse of an index patient, does not seem to be higher than chance, indicating that shared environmental exposure does not seem to be a risk factor in this context. Interestingly, the risk for children of conjugal pairs does seem to be significantly increased (5.8%) in comparison with that of children of pairings with only one affected parent (1.8%). This finding indicates that a "double exposure" or concentration of presumed genetic or environmental susceptibility factors in parents increases MS risk in offspring.[313]

- *Racial clustering.* MS is especially common in persons of Northern European Caucasian stock, particularly those of Nordic extraction. In this regard, it has been hypothesized that the genetic susceptibility to MS developed as a result of genes disseminated during the migration of the Vikings,[296] which may in part account for the latitude effect in Europe. By contrast, different racial groups, such as African blacks, Orientals, Lapps, American Indians, and others appear to be relatively resistant to MS.

- *Candidate genes for multiple sclerosis.* Intensive studies of putative genes with a logical or

TABLE 2.1 — AGE-ADJUSTED RISK OF MULTIPLE SCLEROSIS*

Relationship†	Study Population	MS Risk (%)	Comments
General population	Flemish[1]	0.088	Prevalence ≈1/1000 in northern Caucasian populations
First cousin	Flemish[1]	0.44	Prevalence ≈1/100 or higher in relatives
Aunt/uncle	Flemish	0.66	
Parent	Flemish	1.61	
Child	Flemish	1.73	
Sibling	Flemish	2.10	
Adopted child	Canadian[2]	<0.2	No multiple sclerosis observed in 386 adopted children
Biological child	Canadian	2.70	Risk appears to be associated with genes, not shared environment
Half-sibling	Canadian[3]	1.32	
Sibling	Canadian	3.46	Increased risk linked to degree of genetic identity
Dizygotic twins	Caucasian series[4]	2-5	Range reported in several large studies
Monozygotic twins	Caucasian series	25-30	Strong genetic risk; incomplete penetrance

Representative studies are shown as indicated. All populations are from the high-risk Northern European Caucasian group. When a given risk category (eg, parent) was examined in different study populations, roughly comparable results were found. For the sake of simplicity and because of minor variations in methods, study populations, and results, only comparisons within one representative survey are shown, grouped together; please see original reviews and references for details and additional investigations.

* Age-adjusted risk of multiple sclerosis, taking into account the age structure of the study population and age-of-onset distribution for affected members. The lifetime risk is estimated to be approximately twice the age-adjusted risk determined during the observation period.[61]

† Relationship to MS index cases.

[1]Reference 61, [2]Reference 102, [3]Reference 325, and [4]reviewed in Reference 266.

suspected relation to MS have been disappointing. One exception has been the major histocompatibility (MHC) gene serologically defined as DR2 haplotype (molecular designation, HLA-DRB1*1501-DQA1*0102-DQB1*0602), which has been consistently associated with MS risk in Northern European Caucasians.[266] The magnitude of this effect is thought to be about 5% to 10% of the total genetic risk of MS, although it is not known if the risk is contributed by MHC genes themselves or via nearby linked genes. About 25% of multiplex families show no association with DRB1*1501, suggesting that MS may be genetically heterogeneous. A recent report shows a tight correlation of a point mutation in the RTPRC gene and MS in three families.[172] The PTPRC gene product (also known as CD45) is a receptor protein found on T and B cells and plays an important role in mediation of signaling during cell-to-cell contact in the immune system. Thus it is possible that aberrant forms of this molecule may predispose to disordered immune regulation in MS.

- *Whole genome screens.* Four studies using informative families and microsatellite markers to determine linkage to MS (United States, United Kingdom, Canada, and Finland)[266] have identified approximately 60 regions of the human genome with potential relevance to MS; 10 to 15 of these sites appear particularly promising because of linkage strength and agreement between different research groups. Also, approximately 95% of the genome can be excluded from consideration for a gene of major effect.[64] Obviously, a major research effort will be required to reconcile current findings and fine map regions strongly linked to MS risk.

It should be noted that to date the remarkable advances in human molecular genetics have been limited to diseases caused by single gene defects; no polygenic human condition can yet be said to have been "solved," despite some progress in conditions such as diabetes. However, insights gained from experimental animal models, such as genetic reconstitution in mouse strains with lupus erythematosus immunopathology, may provide insights and strategies with relevance to human polygenic diseases.[243]

Oksenberg and colleagues have recently summarized this vast and exciting body of work.[266] They propose the following model to account for the genetic complexity of MS:

> *The genetic component of MS etiology is believed to result from the action of several genes of moderate effect. The incomplete penetrance of MS susceptibility alleles probably reflects interactions with other genes, posttranscriptional regulatory mechanisms, and significant nutritional and environmental influences. Equally significant, it is also likely that genetic heterogeneity exists, meaning that specific genes influence susceptibility and pathogenesis in some affects but not in others... much of the genetic effect in MS remains to be explained... [identification of specific genes] is likely to define the basic etiology of the disease, improve risk assessment, and influence therapeutics.*

Synthesis of Current Research

Despite the vast amount of the research summarized above and the substantial advances achieved to date, daunting problems remain with regard to complete and compelling explanations of MS epidemiology and genetics. Major issues include at least the following:

- The relative roles of environmental and inherited factors are unknown. For example, the observed concordance rate of MS of 25% to 30% in MZ twins could imply that the relevant susceptibility genes are very important but not completely determinative of disease; thus an environmental trigger or influence seems necessary. Specifically, it appears more likely that a putative environmental agent for MS is (1) an ubiquitous agent (eg, a common virus) causing disease in rare, particularly susceptible individuals, not (2) a unique, uncommon environmental factor (eg, *the* MS virus), which is highly pathogenic in the normal person unlucky enough to be exposed.[73] (Alternatively, it is possible that disease completely depends on stochastic gene interactions or transcription patterns, and genetics are sufficient in this sense for MS. In other words, the genetic legacy for MS provides "all the right pieces," but what is critical is the way, perhaps by chance, that these elements are combined and expressed.[143])
- The degree to which MS is heterogeneous is unknown. Possibly the single clinical phenotype we recognize as MS is due to a number of fundamentally different underlying pathophysiologies. For example, if MS is triggered by many viruses, surveys pinpointing any one virus will be problematic due to the diluting effect of other etiologic viruses. Also, to the degree that MS is caused by different sets of genes in different subgroups of patients, it will be increasingly difficult to establish the association of any one gene in MS, given the "noise" of other genes contributing to the complex phenotype.
- Even if MS is an etiologically unitary disease, the absolute numbers of relevant environmental factors and genes are unknown. For example,

mathematical modeling of MS susceptibility by Phillips[290] indicates that the best fit with observed MS risk patterns occurs with approximately 10 to 15 major interacting genes plus a contribution of a large number of minor background genes. Obviously, the larger number of pieces in the etiological puzzle, the more exponentially difficult it will be to uniquely identify each factor contributing to MS.

In essence, the difficulties listed are analogous to an algebraic equation in which the number of unknowns exceeds the number of facts currently available. This noted, the rapid progress of recent years, coupled with the pace of methodological and conceptual advances, raises the realistic possibility that significant breakthroughs may be achieved in the near future.

3 Immunology, Pathogenesis, and Etiology

Autoimmunity and Multiple Sclerosis

The pathology of multiple sclerosis (MS) is characterized by focal infiltrates of lymphocytes and monocytes, associated with tissue damage to myelin, oligodendrocytes, and axons.[356,409] This pathological picture suggests that MS may be an autoimmune disease; ie, a condition in which tolerance to self is broken and a pathological immune attack against host tissues ensues. (It should be recalled that not all inflammatory pathology is necessarily due to autoimmunity in the strict sense. For example, the immune response observed during hepatitis B infection is primarily antiviral, not antiself. Thus the immunopathology of hepatitis B infection is a secondary consequence of a primary response to the virus. This possibility should always be borne in mind, since MS is a *putative*, but as of yet not proven, autoimmune disease.)

Recent reviews[89,200] have aptly summarized features that suspected and established autoimmune diseases share, including:

- A propensity to be either organ-specific or systemic
- A strong genetic basis, often with linkage to the major histocompatibility complex (MHC)
- A complicated pathogenesis, characterized by multiple steps (Figure 3.1 shows the proposed pathogenesis of systemic lupus erythematosus; MS may depend on similar interactions between multiple genes, environmental factors, and internal processes)

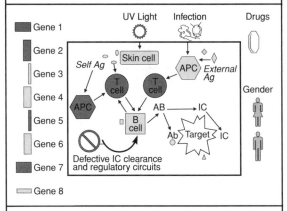

FIGURE 3.1 — POSSIBLE PATHOGENESIS OF SYSTEMIC LUPUS ERYTHEMATOSUS

Abbreviations: AB, antibody; Ag, antigen; APC, antigen-presenting cell; IC, immune complex.

Note multiple environmental factors, modifying genes at each step, and numerous interactions within the host immune system.

Reference 152.

- A disease mechanism that usually is predominantly humoral (eg, in myasthenia gravis) or cell-mediated (eg, type 1 diabetes)
- A suspected environmental trigger, such as a virus or other microorganism
- The fact that an animal model can be induced that mimics the human condition and allows controlled experimental study of pathogenesis and potential treatments.

Immunological aspects of MS[21,273,409] closely follow the general pattern for autoimmunity outlined above. Whether MS is associated with an excess of other autoimmune conditions, over and above what would be expected by chance, is controversial. There is evidence to support modest associations of MS with thyroiditis, uveitis, and perhaps other diseases.[103] The suggestive findings of autoimmune associations in MS should be contrasted with the situation in a florid autoimmune disease such as juvenile diabetes, in which 10% of patients have a second identifiable autoimmune condition.[62]

Animal Models of MS

The most frequently studied animal model for MS is experimental allergic encephalomyelitis (EAE; also designated experimental autoimmune encephalomyelitis in more recent literature). EAE was originally produced by Rivers and colleagues in 1933 by repeated immunization of primates with spinal cord material; since then EAE has been adapted to small laboratory animals, such as inbred mouse strains, and special forms of the model, such as relapsing-remitting EAE, have been formulated.[104] Advances such as transgenic technology have allowed immunologists to study the roles of individual molecules in EAE.[273] In this regard, Owens and colleagues point out a crucial distinction between EAE and MS: whereas in EAE disease can be studied at early states such as susceptibility and initiation, MS patients only come to attention after tissue damage has occurred and symptoms are present, ie, at a much later stage in pathogenesis (Figure 3.2). In any comparison of an experimental model to MS, it is essential to recall the specific step in pathogenesis that is operative. For example, comparing early findings in EAE with late pathology in MS is likely to be misleading.

Because EAE can be transferred by T-cell clones with specificity for myelin antigens, there is general agreement that cellular immunity (most likely CD4 T_H1 cells) is the predominant mediator of immunopathology in this model. EAE has been used successfully to

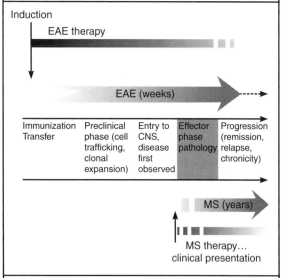

FIGURE 3.2 — COMPARISON OF TREATMENT OF EXPERIMENTAL ALLERGIC ENCEPHALOMYELITIS AND MULTIPLE SCLEROSIS

Induction

EAE therapy

EAE (weeks)

| Immunization Transfer | Preclinical phase (cell trafficking, clonal expansion) | Entry to CNS, disease first observed | Effector phase pathology | Progression (remission, relapse, chronicity) |

MS (years)

MS therapy... clinical presentation

Abbreviations: CNS, central nervous system; EAE, experimental allergic encephalomyelitis; MS, multiple sclerosis.

Some of the discrepancies in results obtained from EAE and MS studies may reflect the fact that many EAE experiments are designed to study the induction phase of disease, whereas MS is studied after disease induction, as its cause is unknown.

Reference 273.

screen potential treatments, although it appears that the animal model is much more susceptible to therapeutic suppression than is MS itself; that is, many of the drugs that are of benefit in EAE are ineffective in MS.

Other animal models of MS are induced by toxins or viruses (eg, Theiler's murine encephalomyelitis virus, mouse hepatitis virus, Semliki Forest virus, and others).[164,179,183,209] It is instructive to recall that most veterinary demyelinating diseases and several human demyelinating diseases are caused by viruses. Thus the ability of viruses to induce immunopathology and demyelination in nature is not in doubt; the relevant question is whether this happens in MS and, if so, what agents and mechanisms are operative. Despite extensive investigations, to date no virus or other microbe has been conclusively linked to MS etiology.

Molecular Immunology and Pathogenesis of Multiple Sclerosis

A vast literature describes the study of virtually every known immunological process as it pertains to MS. Bar-Or and colleagues[21] have provided an insightful guide to this complex topic by extracting five major or central immunological themes, roughly corresponding to key steps in the probable pathophysiology of MS (Figure 3.3):

- Autoreactive T cells in normal individuals and in MS patients with specificity for myelin and other neuroantigens. While autoreactive T cells are found in both populations, there is evidence suggesting that autoreactive T cells in MS patients may be in an enhanced state of activation.
- The selective expression in MS of molecules such as chemokines (chemoattractants such as MCP-1 and RANTES), endothelial adhesion molecules (eg, ICAM-1 and VCAM-1), and matrix metalloproteinases (eg, MMP-9, which degrades extracellular matrix). There is evidence that these molecules are up-regulated in MS and thus may contribute to immune cell invasion into active central nervous system (CNS) lesions.

FIGURE 3.3 — A MODEL OF MULTIPLE SCLEROSIS PATHOPHYSIOLOGY

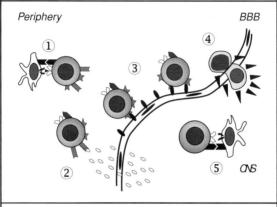

A model of the molecular pathogenesis of multiple sclerosis (MS): 1) myelin autoreactive T-cell activation in the periphery; 2) chemoattraction of activated cells to central nervous system (CNS) mediated by chemokine/chemokine receptor interactions; 3) adhesion of activated cells to blood–brain-barrier (BBB) endothelium via adhesion molecules and their receptors; 4) matrix metalloproteinase release facilitates infiltration of activated cells across BBB basement membrane and into CNS parenchyma; 5) reactivation of autopathogenic cells in CNS mediates damage to myelin and axonal injury.

Reference 21.

- Role of the B7-costimulatory pathway. The B7 class of molecules are expressed on antigen presenting cells (APCs), which subsequently react with T cells. Depending on the means by which APCs interact with T cells, the latter are either activated or made anergic. There is evidence that specific patterns of B7 molecule expression on APCs occur in MS and may therefore lead to selective costimulation and thus increased T-cell reactivity.

- Proinflammatory cytokines in MS. Cytokines are soluble molecules that influence the activity of the immune system. Together with specific subsets of immune cells such as type 1 helper T cells (T_H1) and type 2 helper T cells (T_H2), cytokines form a complex, interactive network that influences the state of the immune system. A simplified, but useful, view of the immune system considers two polar responses, (1) a proinflammantory state with active cellular immunity or (2) a less inflammatory, more humorally mediated state of reactivity. Most studies of MS to date favor the first pattern, with prominence of cytokines such as tumor necrosis factor (TNF)-α and interleukin (IL)-12, as well as the T_H1 subset of helper cells, all of which are proinflammatory and would be expected to provide stimulation to effector cells such as macrophages and microglia.
- Role of molecular mimicry. There is evidence that some microbial antigens may resemble or mimic myelin epitopes at the molecular level. Thus initial protective host responses directed against infecting microbes could secondarily result in pathologic cross-reactive immune responses that damage normal tissues, such as myelin.

In addition to the many studies implicating cellular immunity in MS, other investigations have indicated that humoral immunity may play an important role in pathogenesis. MS is characterized by an increase of immunoglobulin synthesis within the CNS. In >90% of patients with established MS, electrophoresis of cerebrospinal fluid antibodies shows discrete bands, an oligoclonal pattern. A major research goal[272] has been to determine the specificity or target of these antibodies, since in conditions such as CNS infections where the inciting agent is known, eg, subacute sclerosing panencephalitis due to measles virus, a substantial portion of the immunoglobulin is directed against the inciting agent.[407] In an ingenious set of experiments Williamson and colleagues[407] characterized the immunoglobulin G (IgG) repertoire from active plaque and periplaque regions in two MS brains and determined that antibody responses were highly restricted and also directed against DNA, suggesting a link to other similar autoimmune diseases that affect the CNS, such as systemic lupus erythematosus. These dramatic and important findings, if confirmed, could be a crucial step in defining the etiology of MS.

One inevitable difficulty in interpreting the immunological findings above is establishing causality, that is, distinguishing primary events from secondary phenomena. Thus, as shown in Figure 3.4, tissue damage may elicit immune responses, and immune responses may elicit tissue damage. Without prior knowledge of the inciting event or etiology, it is difficult to differentiate these two possibilities (eg, to know if antimyelin T cells are the cause or effect of demyeli-

---

FIGURE 3.4 — DILEMMA OF CAUSATION:
"THE CHICKEN AND THE EGG"

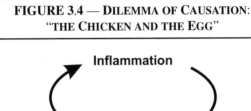

Inflammation

Tissue Damage

Determining causality of multiple sclerosis from immunological findings is difficult. Just as in the question "Which came first: the chicken or the egg?" it is difficult to assess whether inflammation causes tissue damage or vice versa.

nation). After stroke and other destructive lesions of the CNS, eg, antimyelin responses are well-documented. Perhaps the strongest, most direct argument in favor of the primacy of immune phenomena in MS pathogenesis is the success achieved with medications designed to favorably address immunopathology. Only with better understanding of the cause and sequence of MS pathogenesis will it be possible to definitively resolve these issues.

Etiology

Despite the impressive advances in pathology, genetics, and immunology noted, currently the etiology of MS is unknown. If the study of MS could be fixed or anchored to a definite inciting cause, the pace of progress focused on the prevention or cure of MS would be accelerated dramatically.

Possibly the biological jigsaw puzzle of MS will be solved piecemeal, eg, by the gradual, sequential identification of 10 genes that are pathogenic. Alternatively, the identification of a key piece in the puzzle may illuminate all the rest, eg, the unequivocal demonstration of an environmental trigger for MS. Perhaps progress will even depend on discovering a fundamentally new biological theory or process, eg, a breakthrough in one autoimmune disease that will lead to the understanding of all other autoimmune diseases.

Any complete theory of MS will have to account for the characteristic dissemination of demyelination in *particular* space and time parameters. All physicians caring for MS patients are struck by how clinically stable most patients appear between attacks. It is as if the clinical seas are calm for a prolonged period; an immunological storm then suddenly occurs with a specific location, onset, and duration; and, finally, recovery and stability ensue for months or years. Why, for example, does patient Smith develop a new lesion in the right frontal lobe white matter on January 10th? Why not her pons, or March 6th? Why does she return to baseline status in 3 weeks, instead of 6 weeks? Why was she completely asymptomatic for 6 months before and after this attack?

Clearly, any global explanation (eg, the general tendency toward antimyelin autoimmunity) does not address the distinctive, punctuated pattern that characterizes many patients, especially early in relapsing-remitting MS (RRMS). Conceivably, identification and control of the proximal, immediate cause of MS exacerbations could lead to clinical improvement, even if the underlying or first cause of MS has not been identified or addressed. From the perspective of pathology, Sobel[356] observes:

> *The reason for these typical patterns of lesion location are not known but may relate to distinct microenvironments in these sites. The proximity to flow of cerebrospinal fluid or features of their vascular perfusion might result in high concentrations of circulating inflammatory mediators or plasma proteins in these areas [optic nerves, periventricular white matter, subpial brain stem, spinal cord] . Alternatively, there might be subtle, as yet unidentified intrinsic differences in the composition of the myelin or the extracellular matrix in these areas.*

In the JHM coronavirus model of MS in mice, our laboratory has found that plaques of demyelination appear when and where viral replication occurs in white matter. Presumably, activity of the JHM virus at a given site leads to increased local viral antigen expression, chemokine liberation, and tissue invasion by immune cells.[391] Thus a plaque of focal demyelination in a specific location and time occurs. If this animal model is relevant to plaque development in MS, perhaps similar changes can be observed in MS tissue by serial MRI scans, providing a clue as to why normal appearing white matter is transformed into an early plaque. Perhaps MS relapses are like the conjunction of two planets, a situation in which lesion formation depends on the stochastic alignment of local and systemic immune responses at the same time and place. In this regard, Martino and colleagues[226] have formulated a dual-signal hypothesis for MS in which they propose that two concomitant, but possibly unrelated, inflammatory events, one in the CNS and one in the periphery, interact to trigger attacks and sustain immunopathology.

4   Neuroimaging

Typical MRI Findings in Multiple Sclerosis

The advent of nuclear magnetic resonance imaging (MRI) has transformed investigation of patients with multiple sclerosis, both in terms of clinical practice and research. MRI thus is the neuroimaging modality of choice in suspected and established multiple sclerosis.

In most applications, MRI scanning depends on the physicochemical environment of water protons in the brain and spinal cord.[233,279] Different operator-selectable instructions are programmed into the scanner in order to obtain MRI sequences that optimally demonstrate typical findings in multiple sclerosis (MS) as illustrated in Figure 4.1. The most common abnormalities noted during conventional MRI scanning in MS are T2-intense foci in white matter (Figure 4.1C), sometimes informally referred to as unidentified bright objects (UBOs). Other sequences also may be very informative; for example, T2-weighted sequences done with free-water suppression techniques (eg, fluid attenuated inversion recovery [FLAIR]) improve the conspicuity of lesions, particularly at the margins of ventricles (Figure 4.1E). Radiological:pathological correlation studies have shown excellent correspondence between the observed areas of abnormal MRI signal and tissue lesions. On the other hand, MRI abnormalities usually do not have a precise histological correlate; thus T2 hyperintensities are thought to result from changes in the environment of water molecules consequent to a complex combination of pro-

FIGURE 4.1 — DIFFERENT MRI SEQUENCES IN TYPICAL MS

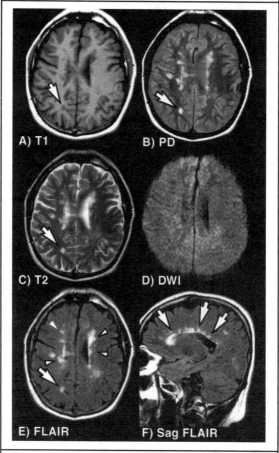

A) T1 B) PD C) T2 D) DWI E) FLAIR F) Sag FLAIR

Magnetic resonance imaging (MRI) techniques which are commonly used to image multiple sclerosis (MS) lesions are shown. The patient imaged is a 38-year-old man who has had relapsing-remitting MS (RRMS) for 10 years. At the time of the MRI study, he did not have any active or new lesions. In views *A* through *E*, transverse sections are shown to illustrate the typical appearance of lesions (chronic demyelinated plaques), cerebrospinal fluid

(CSF), and white matter in each MRI sequence. A typical juxtacortical (gray-white junction involving U fibers) lesion is marked by an arrow in views *A* through *E*; in addition, numerous other MS lesions are shown, especially in a periventricular location (arrowheads in view *E*). View F represents a sagittal orientation.

A) T1-Weighted MRI: Note that the marked juxtacortical lesion *(arrow)* appears hypointense by this technique; such lesions are often referred to as "black holes" and may represent areas of white matter destruction.

B) Proton Density (PD) MRI: Because CSF is light gray and MS lesions are bright white *(arrow),* periventricular lesions are easily distinguished from the CSF in the lateral ventricles by this technique.

C) T2-Weighted MRI: Both CSF and MS lesions appear bright white on T2-weighted MRI scans. While the T2 intense (T2I) lesions are typical of MS and dramatically demonstrated by this technique, periventricular lesions may be difficult to distinguish from ventricular CSF in T2-weighted MRI studies.

D) Diffusion-Weighted Imaging (DWI) MRI: This technique reflects alterations in micromolecular water motion and is particularly useful in detecting abnormalities during acute ischemia or demyelination. Because the patient was stable at the time of this study, without any new or active lesions, his DWI scan is normal. Active MS lesions appear as bright white areas on DWI (not shown) and gadolinium infusion studies (Figure 4.2, Criterion 1).

E) Fluid Attenuated Inversion Recovery (FLAIR) MRI: In this technique, free-water signals are suppressed; therefore CSF appears black, and bright white lesions of MS are conspicuous and readily distinguished from ventricular CSF. In addition to the juxtacortical lesion shown by an *arrow,* periventricular lesions are noted by *arrowheads*.

F) Sagittal FLAIR MRI: The technique is identical to that performed with view E, except that the section is oriented to show the midsagittal plane. Typical of MS are lesions *(arrows)* which prominently involve the corpus callosum, often extending perpendicularly from this white matter structure.

Images provided by Dr. Howard Rowley

cesses, including edema, loss of cells, demyelination, and inflammation.

What is the utility of MRI in clinical practice? To answer this question, it is convenient to consider MRI in two very different circumstances: when MS is suspected and after the diagnosis of MS has been established.

Application of MRI in Suspected or Early Multiple Sclerosis

For persons with initial symptoms suggestive of MS, the main concerns are diagnosis and prognosis. From the patient's perspective, the important questions are, Will I develop MS? Am I likely to be disabled? Of course, definitive answers to these questions, the "gold standard," can only come from clinical assessments at a later date. In terms of initial MRI studies, however, the relevant issue is how well radiological findings at onset will predict eventual clinical course. As indicated below, it turns out that MRI is highly predictive in this context.

Several large investigations have addressed the predictive contribution of MRI to suspected MS, usually in the context of clinically isolated syndromes (CIS) suggestive of MS, such as a well-defined first attack of optic neuritis, brain stem dysfunction, or spinal cord deficits. The set of patients with CIS is not identical to the entire population of patients who will be evaluated for possible MS, some of whom will have insidious or nonspecific presentations. Nonetheless, the best studies of MRI predictive value have been performed in the CIS group, and it is reasonable to assume that the findings in CIS patients are applicable to other patients with suspected MS.

As shown in Table 4.1, head MRI findings at first presentation in CIS patients are highly predictive of eventual development of MS. It is remarkable that these studies, performed in different patient populations and by means of different methodologies, should have very similar findings. Specifically, a normal MRI is very informative and indicates that the chance of developing MS is only about 10% at 10-year follow-up; that is, the negative predictive value (NPV) of MRI is quite high in this setting. On the other hand, the positive predictive value (PPV) of an abnormal MRI with a "demyelinating" appearance is estimated to be only 40% to 50% over the intermediate term (2 to 3 years) and moderately higher if follow-up is extended to 10 years. Thus head MRI scans showing suggestive abnormalities will identify most patients who develop definite MS, as well as a significant number of patients who apparently will never develop MS. In a mathematical analysis, Barkof and colleagues[22] have shown that there is a trade-off between MRI sensitivity versus specificity as a function of the minimal number of characteristic lesions required to consider a scan abnormal. For example, if only one lesion is chosen as the criterion for abnormality, the approximate MRI sensitivity for eventual MS conversion is 95%, while specificity is only 50%; at the other extreme, if identification of ≥ 9 lesions is taken as the criterion for an abnormal scan, sensitivity falls to 40% but specificity rises to 90%.

Investigators have proposed sets of criteria that optimize head MRI sensitivity and specificity with regard to prediction of eventual MS; MRI findings that have proven reliable in prospective studies[378] include gadolinium-enhancing lesions, ≥ 9 or more T2-intense lesions, and lesions in an infratentorial (posterior fossa), juxtacortical (gray-white junction), or periventricular location (Figure 4.2). These MRI features have recently been incorporated into formal criteria for the diagnosis of MS.[234] In the study of Barkhof and associates,[22] 50% of patients who converted from CIS to clinically definite MS did so at ≤ 9 months, and

TABLE 4.1 — PERCENTAGE OF PATIENTS WITH CIS CONVERTING TO CLINICALLY DEFINITE MS AS A FUNCTION OF NUMBER OF MRI LESIONS ON INITIAL MRI AND LENGTH OF FOLLOW-UP

Reference	Jacobs[171]	ONSG[270]			Soderstrom[357]		Morrissey[245], O'Riordan[263]					Barkhof[22]	
Patient type	CIS	ON			CIS		CIS					CIS	
# of MRI lesions*	≥2	0	1-2	≥3	0-2	≥3	0	1	2-3	4-10	>10	0	≥1
Years follow-up†													
1	12	3	15	25	5	50	—	—	—	—	—	0	—
2	38	5	29	30	10	60	—	—	—	—	—	—	—
3	50	10	26	38	15	75	—	—	—	—	—	8	54
5	—	16	37	51	—	—	6	17	67	92	80	—	—
10	—	—	—	—	—	—	11	33	87	87‡	85	—	—

Abbreviations: CIS, clinically isolated syndromes [suggestive of demyelination]; MRI, magnetic resonance imaging; ON, optic neuritis; ONSG, Optic Neuritis Study Group.

* Number of lesions seen on standard head MRI and considered characteristic of multiple sclerosis.

† Years after initial episode; percentages of patients manifesting a second attack, indicative of clinically definite multiple sclerosis are indicated. Please see original references for exact criteria applied in each study.

‡ The apparent fall from 92% at 5 years to 87% at 10 years is due to variation in the remaining cohort because of patient dropout.

References 22, 171, 245, 263, 270, 357.

FIGURE 4.2 — MRI FEATURES WITH HIGH SENSITIVITY AND SPECIFICITY FOR MS

At least three of the following four criteria must be met:

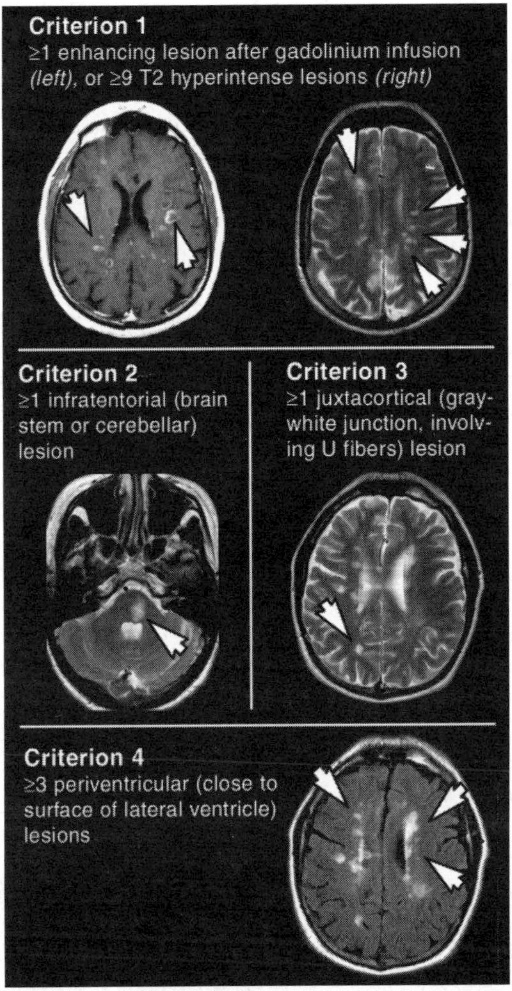

Criterion 1
≥1 enhancing lesion after gadolinium infusion *(left)*, or ≥9 T2 hyperintense lesions *(right)*

Criterion 2
≥1 infratentorial (brain stem or cerebellar) lesion

Criterion 3
≥1 juxtacortical (gray-white junction, involving U fibers) lesion

Criterion 4
≥3 periventricular (close to surface of lateral ventricle) lesions

MRI criteria derived from References 22 and 378, and incorporated into the guidelines of the McDonald Committee, Reference 234.

Images provided by Dr. Howard Rowley.

90% of converting patients did so by 30 months. Thus development of MS tends to occur quickly after initial symptoms, and nonconversion in the first few years of observation is a relatively good prognostic sign. Barkhof and colleagues[22] suggested that in the context of suspected MS, specificity of MRI is more important than sensitivity, since <50% of CIS patients convert to MS. In other words, since the population under consideration has a substantial number of subjects who will not develop disease, the most likely and troublesome potential error is that of false-positive prediction of MS.

Brex and colleagues[46] showed that a follow-up head MRI performed ≥ 3 months after the initial scan may provide useful additional prognostic information, especially if new lesions (MRI equivalents of attacks that are disseminated in time and space) are observed. Thus 55% of patients with new lesions on follow-up MRI eventually developed MS; in contrast, only 5% of patients with stable repeat MRI scans developed MS after 1 year of follow-up. The findings of Barkhof and Brex and their associates may provide useful guidance with regard to the possibility of early treatment with MS-modifying agents. In this context, many authorities have advocated administration of disease-modifying treatment early in the course of MS; on the other hand, such treatment obviously is contraindicated in the large number of subjects who never develop MS. A simple resolution of this dilemma may be as follows: since both clinical and MRI conversion are likely to occur early in the course of patients "destined" to develop MS, in ambiguous cases, merely waiting 3 to 6 months for a repeat head MRI will provide information to differentiate individuals in whom MS development is likely or unlikely.

In addition to predicting conversion to MS, are there MRI features at presentation that are predictive of the likely severity of eventual MS, ie, the prognosis for individual patients? This issue has been investigated by many groups, most notably by O'Riordan and colleagues,[263] who conducted a 10-year prospective study (Table 4.2). These investigators found that prognosis was good for many patients, especially in those with a small number of lesions on initial head MRI, most of whom had little serious disability at study end. On the other hand, an active MRI scan at onset (eg, >2 to 3 typical lesions) tended to be associated with increased risk of significant disability, secondary progressive course, and continued development of new lesions on subsequent MRI. Remarkably, of the 81 patients in the CIS cohort followed for 10 years, 57 had relatively good outcomes such as continued CIS, possible-probable MS, or benign MS, with median Expanded Disability Status Scores (EDSS) of 1, 2, and 2 respectively (see Table 4.2 footnote for explanation). This result indicates the generally favorable outlook in a representative patient population of patients with CIS or suspected MS. The possibility that individuals may be exceptions to the general rules above should always be kept in mind and appropriate caution expressed during patient counseling. Currently, MRI prognostication is being reinvestigated in the context of new MRI techniques (eg, FLAIR, atrophy measures) and with regard to the implications for early treatment with disease-modifying medications.

In summary, a reasonably strong and positive answer can be given to the question of MRI prediction of the likelihood and severity of eventual MS.

- A normal head MRI (ie, no significant lesions suggestive of MS) signifies a very small chance of evolution to clinically definite MS; in the few cases in which MS does develop, disease course is usually benign.
- An active head MRI (eg, 5 to 10 lesions suggestive of MS) indicates a high risk of conver-

TABLE 4.2 — PREDICTION OF TYPE OF MS AND EXTENT OF DISABILITY BASED ON INITIAL MRI IN PATIENTS WITH CIS SUGGESTIVE OF POSSIBLE MS (10-YEAR FOLLOW-UP)

Initial MRI	Outcome (10 years)
Normal	11% eventual conversion to CDMS MS benign (EDSS ≤3) in all cases
2-3 lesions	87% eventual conversion to CDMS only 13% of patients have EDSS >5.5
>10 lesions	85% eventual conversion to CDMS 35% of patients have EDSS >5.5)

Final Disease Type, 10 years *(EDSS, median and range)*	Initial MRI *(No. of lesions, median and range)*
Benign 2 (0-3)	3 (0-74)
Relapsing-remitting 4 (3.5-6)	13 (2-31)
Secondary-progressive 6.5 (4-10)	18 (2-29)

Abbreviations: CDMS, clinically definite multiple sclerosis; CIS, clinically isolated syndromes; EDSS, expanded disability status scale; MRI, magnetic resonance imaging; MS, multiple sclerosis

EDSS values: where 0 is normal and 10 is dead due to MS. EDSS grade 5.5 indicates ambulatory limit without aid or rest of 100 meters.

Adapted from Reference 263. Recently, an update of this cohort with mean follow-up of 14.1 years has been reported (Reference 418).

sion to definite MS, and the disease course may be moderate or severe.

- Intermediate results on head MRI appear less predictive but may indicate an intermediate or variable course. Depending on patient characteristics, a more extensive workup than usual, including analysis of cerebrospinal fluid (CSF), evoked potentials, repeat head MRI, spinal MRI, and other tests may be indicated for delineation of diagnosis and prognosis in patients in whom initial MRI scans show intermediate levels of activity (see Chapter 5, *Diagnosis and Differential Diagnosis*) .

In cases presenting with symptoms and signs referable to the spinal cord, clearly MRI should be directed to this site (Figure 4.3), although head MRI remains informative with regard to the prediction of eventual MS.

4

Application of MRI in Established Multiple Sclerosis

In addition to the application of MRI in initial, suspected MS, research has shown that MRI is also very informative in patients with established disease. For example, most large studies employing state-of-the-art head MRI have shown characteristic abnormalities in >95% of patients with definite MS[188]; in the minority of patients in whom MS appears established on clinical grounds but head MRI is normal, spinal MRI will usually show typical lesions.

The criteria for optimal MRI sensitivity and specificity (Figure 4.2) have been applied to established MS, as well as suspected MS. In general, the power of these criteria has been very robust, correctly identifying MS and correctly excluding other conditions, such as cerebrovascular disease. Nonetheless, certain conditions resemble MS clinically and on occasion may have similar or identical MRI appearances (see Chapter 5). From this it follows that MRI alone can never achieve 100% specificity, especially when the population under study involves a substantial number of patients with conditions that may mimic MS.

Since MRI is an accurate, but not perfect, reflection of the underlying pathology of MS, it was hoped that MRI measures could serve as surrogate indicators

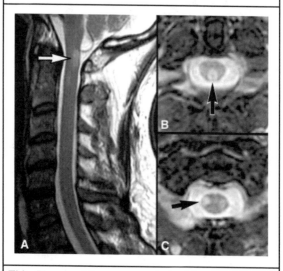
of disease status, analogous to the chest radiograph in pneumonia or serum creatinine in renal failure. Unfortunately, this has not turned out to be the case, at least not with standard MRI procedures in current use. For example, an analysis by van Walderveen and Barkhof[389] showed that the average correlation coefficient between the burden of T2 lesions on head MRI and EDSS in nine large studies was 0.31, a value that

most statisticians would regard as showing little or perhaps no meaningful relationship between the measures. Certainly, at the level of an individual patient, correlation between MRI and clinical status is problematic, as illustrated in Figure 4.4. In part, the poor correlation of MRI and disability may be addressed with advances in MRI technique and with better measures of clinical disability. Nevertheless, intractable problems are likely to remain to some extent, including the impact of undetected, microscopic disease in normal white matter and the fact that certain areas of the central nervous system are unusually eloquent (eg, optic nerve, spinal cord), and lesions in these sites may disproportionately contribute to disability.

Longitudinal investigations, in which MRI scans were done at frequent intervals, have revealed that MS is surprisingly active and dynamic radiologically, particularly during the early stages of disease. For example, most studies have shown that the number of new gadolinium-enhancing MRI lesions observed is approximately 5 to 10 times the number of clinical attacks or symptomatic events noted in the same time period. Figure 4.5 shows the monthly findings in one individual and indicates that MRI events are frequent and correlate poorly with disability level, particularly during the early stages of mild relapsing-remitting MS (RRMS). Parenthetically, the example also indicates that a random, "spot check" MRI would likely be misleading; that is, the high level of variation in MRI activity between months implies that any one observation would be unlikely to accurately reflect the complex allover pattern revealed by frequent sampling.

Other investigations have attempted to determine if there is a relationship between MRI features and the clinical subtypes of MS. For the most part, there is substantial overlap between RRMS and secondary-progressive MS (SPMS), with a trend for greater T2 lesion burden and greater volume of T1 hypointense le-

FIGURE 4.4 — LACK OF CORRELATION BETWEEN MAGNETIC RESONANCE IMAGING AND MEASURES OF CLINICAL DISABILITY

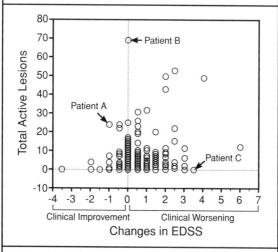

In this study, 281 multiple sclerosis (MS) patients underwent clinical assessment (expanded disability status scale [EDSS]) and head magnetic resonance imaging (MRI) scans at 1) baseline and 2) 24 to 36 months later. Patients were recruited from four large centers and included all MS subtypes and degrees of disability; 41% of patients received disease-modifying treatment. The figure above displays the change in clinical status plotted against the total number of new or enhancing lesions observed on the follow-up scan. Intuitively, one would expect that patients with more active scans at follow-up would have worsening clinical disease when compared with patients whose MRI scans were quiescent. A weak association of scan activity with worsening disease was noted (correlation coefficient 0.13, $P = 0.02$). This correlation is meaningful when comparing groups of patients (eg, as in the arms of a clinical trial), but may be unreliable in the case of individual patients. For example, consider the marked patients: Patient A (1.0 EDSS point improved, 25 active lesions), Patient B (clinically unchanged, 70 active lesions), and Patient C clinically worse by 3.5 EDSS points, no active lesions).

Adapted from: Reference 118.

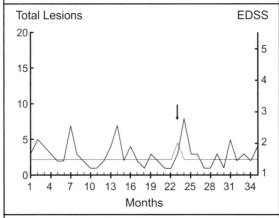

FIGURE 4.5 — MONTHLY MAGNETIC RESONANCE IMAGING

Shown are the results of clinical assessments (expanded disability status scale [EDSS], dotted line) and MRI determinations (total active, or gadolinium-enhancing, lesions per scan, solid line) for an individual patient studied at monthly intervals. Note the pattern typical of most patients with early, mild relapsing-remitting MS, ie, active or ongoing disease as measured by MRI but few clinical attacks or exacerbations. Thus the only event to reach the threshold of clinical detection was a minor exacerbation noted at 23 months (arrow). Individual patients vary widely in terms of clinical and MRI patterns (see Smith 1993), but in most instances, MRI occurrences vastly outnumber clinical attacks.

Adapted from: Reference 354.

sions in the latter. Primary-progressive MS (PPMS) tends to have fewer gadolinium-enhancing lesions and less T2 lesion burden, in comparison with RRMS and SPMS.[350] Little MRI data exist on progressive-relapsing MS (PRMS); this subtype may be biologically indistinguishable from PPMS. Thus, at least by standard MRI measures, these differences are not sufficiently significant to allow accurate designation of subtype on MRI appearances alone.

What conclusions, then, may be reached concerning the role of MRI in established MS? As it turns out, MRI is obtained less often in established disease than it is in suspected disease, in which the application of MRI is virtually universal. Nevertheless, in the following situations MRI may be very informative in established MS patients:

- *Putative MS with atypical clinical findings or unusual course.* Examples of such patients may include those refractory to treatment, having prominent systemic findings, or manifesting disproportionate or nonanatomical findings that suggest nonorganicity. As indicated, virtually all patients with established MS will have a characteristic head MRI study. Therefore, a normal head MRI calls the diagnosis of MS into question and indicates the need for thorough reassessment. As indicated, in the few MS patients with a normal head MRI, spinal MRI and CSF evaluations are usually abnormal. In some cases, an extensive differential diagnosis (see Chapter 5) may need to be considered.

- *Monitoring of disease activity.* As indicated, *repeat MRI scanning on a routine basis may be misleading and is not likely to assist management in the majority of patients with established MS*, since the correlation of MRI with current disability is poor. However, careful application of repeat MRI studies to *selected* patients may be of value. For example, a patient with definite, but mild, RRMS may be psychologically "on the fence" with regard to the decision to initiate or delay disease-modifying treatment. While it is important to treat the patient on the basis of the entire clinical presentation ("treat the patient, not the scan"), relying only on the informed judgment of patient and physician, at times the MRI may have significant impact on these judgments. Hypothetically, an MRI study repeated in 6 to 12 months with gadolinium contrast may either be unchanged or may show evidence of florid, active subclinical disease. While there is no hard evidence to indicate that the follow-up scan conclusively indicates prognosis for an individual patient, certainly either MRI result (stable or active) would be informative and worth taking into consideration.

- *Correlation of head and spinal MRI.* Some patients with established MS may benefit from comparison of MRI scans at these two sites. For example, at times MS and vascular conditions may have similar head MRI appearances. However, most primary vascular disorders affecting the brain do not affect the spinal cord; thus typical lesions disseminated to both spinal cord and brain strongly favor MS. By contrast, in patients presenting with a spinal cord syndrome, a spinal MRI may be compatible with either an isolated local process, such as glioma, or with MS. If white matter lesions are seen on head MRI, demonstration of disseminated disease in this case indicates the presence of MS or a similar condition and may spare the patient invasive procedures such as biopsy.

- *Research applications.* While currently impractical for routine clinical use, serial (eg, monthly) MRI scans have served as useful surrogate measures of disease activity in both exploratory and definitive clinical trials. Also, advanced and research MRI techniques, discussed in the next section, offer the promise of improved clinical correlation and may be added to the standard assessment of established patients in the future.

Advanced and Research Applications of Neuroimaging to Multiple Sclerosis

While conventional MRI (Figure 4.1) is sufficient for the management of most patients with MS, virtually every neuroimaging modality has been applied to MS in special clinical circumstances or in research applications. For example, patients with retained metal fragments or other contraindications to MRI are usually evaluated by computerized tomography (CT) scanning. In MS, head CT may reveal low-density foci in the periventicular, cerebellar, brain stem white matter, and active lesions may enhance after contrast administration. Nevertheless, the sensitivity and detail of white matter pathology seen on CT is less prominent than on MRI, which ordinarily is the preferred procedure. A normal head MRI is unusual in MS and calls the diagnosis into question, whereas normal head CT studies are not unusual in early MS.

Although spinal MRI has good sensitivity for MS lesions and usually will rule out other pathologies, occasionally myelography or combined CT-myelography may be required, eg, to evaluate superimposed compressive lesions. Rarely, spinal angiography may be necessary to evaluate possible spinal vascular malformations, although in the future spinal magnetic resonance angiography (MRA) may have sufficient sensitivity to replace conventional angiography. Similarly, head MRA or catheter angiography may be required if vascular conditions such as vasculitis are a serious differential diagnostic concern. MR venography (MRV) is rarely of clinical use in suspected MS, although interestingly, research using high-resolution MRV has confirmed the perivenous nature of most MS plaques.[370] MR spectroscopy (MRS) is a promising research tool that may provide increased histopathological specificity to the study of MS lesions.[16] The principal clinical use of MRS in MS is to distinguish large "tumefactive" MS plaques from neoplasms (Figure 4.6). Typically, neoplasms tend to have marked increases in the MRS choline peak[301] and increased blood flow on perfusion studies, in contrast to the decreases usually seen in MS lesions.[112] Single photon emission computed tomography (SPECT)[265] and positron emission tomography (PET) have also been applied to MS in research settings.[37]

Specialized MRI techniques that may be relevant to clinical practice in the near future include diffusion-weighted imaging (DWI) (Figure 4.1D), which depends on micromolecular water motion; diffusion tensor imaging (DTI), which takes into account the directionality of diffusion properties; perfusion MRI, which reflects blood supply to tissue; magnetization transfer imaging (MTI), reflecting the interaction of water and macromolecules during relaxation of the magnetic resonance; and functional MRI (fMRI), which identifies brain regions activated during specified tasks, such as visual or motor paradigms. Use of DWI and perfusion MRI sequences, for example, may help to distinguish demyelinating diseases from cerebrovascular conditions. Also, MTI and DTI may reveal axonal damage. In addition, automated segmentation and related procedures allow brain regions or lesions to be detected and quantitated by computerized protocols requiring little or no human input. Automated methods may never be relevant to routine clinical use because of artifacts and the need for the judgment of an experienced radiologist; however, for clinical trials and research applications, these techniques may offer the advantages of speed and complete objectivity.

With the increasing recognition that axons are damaged in MS and that axonal loss or other forms of tissue destruction may play a prominent role in permanent disability (see Chapter 3, *Immunology, Pathogenesis, and Etiology*), attention has turned to MRI

FIGURE 4.6 — MAGNETIC RESONANCE SPECTROSCOPY AND DIFFERENTIAL DIAGNOSIS: MULTIPLE SCLEROSIS VS TUMOR

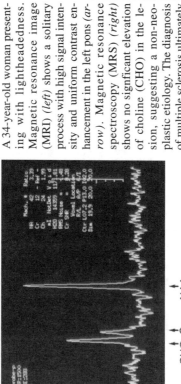
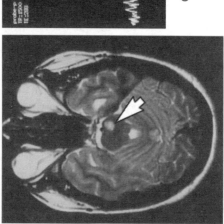

A 34-year-old woman presenting with lightheadedness. Magnetic resonance image (MRI) (*left*) shows a solitary process with high signal intensity and uniform contrast enhancement in the left pons (*arrow*). Magnetic resonance spectroscopy (MRS) (*right*) shows no significant elevation of choline (CHO) in the lesion, suggesting a non-neoplastic etiology. The diagnosis of multiple sclerosis ultimately was made on the basis of additional laboratory testing and clinical observation.

Abbreviations: CHO, choline [peak]; Cr, creatine [peak]; NAA, N-acetyl aspartate [peak].

Images provided by Dr. Victor Haughton

analysis of cerebral atrophy. Research currently is addressing the optimal means of quantitating cerebral atrophy and relating atrophy to the stages of MS, as well as to treatment. Hopefully, in the future, standardized atrophy measures will provide useful guidelines for optimal patient treatment and monitoring.

Summary of MRI in Multiple Sclerosis Management

4

MRI and other neuroimaging modalities have revolutionized the assessment of patients with suspected and established MS. Unless contraindications exist, MRI should be obtained in virtually every patient at onset to clarify diagnosis and provide reliable prognostic information, although the probabilistic nature of this prediction should be remembered when counseling individual patients. MRI is also of utility in special circumstances in established MS, particularly when there are atypical clinical features, difficult therapeutic decisions, or clinical trials of putative new treatments. Undoubtedly, in the near future, research will identify improved neuroimaging modalities, and these advances will be rapidly transferred into routine clinical practice.

Along with the promise of modern neuroimaging comes the danger that it will be used uncritically or inappropriately. For example, neuroradiological authorities such as Trizulzi and Scotti[385] have noted:

It is widely accepted that MRI findings are not totally specific for the diagnosis of multiple sclerosis. White matter lesions that mimic those of multiple sclerosis may be detected in both normal volunteers and patients harboring different diseases. Virtually all the characteristic features of multiple sclerosis are sometimes encountered in other conditions affecting predominantly the white matter... It becomes clear that without fur-

ther clinical information MRI cannot reliably differentiate between different conditions that can lead to white matter multifocal lesions.

Similarly, Charles Poser,[297] a neurologist who has carefully studied the problem of MS diagnosis, observes:

During the past few years, there has been an increasing emphasis on MRI [for diagnosis of multiple sclerosis]... Regrettably, taking the history of the patient's disease has become more and more perfunctory, and is often replaced by interpretation of the MRI films by radiologists who usually receive only limited information about the patient. Many neurologists do not have, or take, the opportunity of reviewing the MRI films themselves and are unaware that many conditions cause MRI appearances that mimic those of MS.

Poser indicates that misdiagnosis has significant consequences. For example, he documents patients with chronic fatigue syndrome, complicated migraine, posttraumatic syndrome, psychiatric diseases, and other conditions who were incorrectly diagnosed as having MS on the basis of uncritical assessment of MRI abnormalities; several of these patients were inappropriately treated with interferon.

In summary, both neuroradiological and neurological experts agree that MRI has made a dramatic, positive contribution to MS diagnosis and management. However, these authorities also point to the real possibility of error if MRI is applied uncritically. The remarkable images and technological glamour of MRI are seductive and may cause the naive or unwary to suppose that a careful history, examination, and discussion with each patient can be dispensed with. In this regard, the excellent MRI analyses provided by colleagues in neuroradiology should not be an excuse for substandard assessment by clinicians.

5

Diagnosis and
Differential Diagnosis

Introduction

Patients in whom multiple sclerosis (MS) is suspected span a wide spectrum of diagnostic difficulty. In many cases, identification of MS is quite straightforward. On the other hand, individual patients with suspected MS may sometimes be among the most diagnostically challenging in neurologic practice. In considering this diagnosis, the author has found it useful to follow the algorithm outlined in Figure 5.1. Essentially, a stratified approach is suggested, and it is usually not difficult to place a patient in one of four categories, each of which has a specific set of diagnostic problems and solutions. Because many patients will have features highly suggestive of MS at presentation, the discussion will first focus on the diagnosis and workup of typical patients (group I), after which atypical or unusual presentations (groups II-IV) will be reviewed.

Group I: Typical Multiple Sclerosis Presentation

In most large prospective series, approximately 30% to 40% of patients suspected of MS will have findings highly supportive of definite MS after initial clinical and neuroimaging assessment. For example, consider the following case: A 25-year-old woman presents to her physician after several attacks consisting of recurrent paresthesias, leg weakness, and monocular visual blurring, with each episode re-

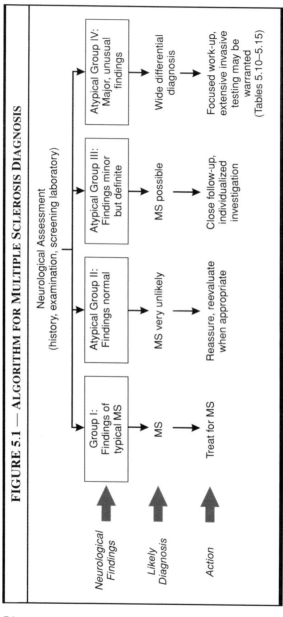

FIGURE 5.1 — ALGORITHM FOR MULTIPLE SCLEROSIS DIAGNOSIS

Neurological Assessment
(history, examination, screening laboratory)

Neurological Findings

| Group I: Findings of typical MS | Atypical Group II: Findings normal | Atypical Group III: Findings minor but definite | Atypical Group IV: Major, unusual findings |

Likely Diagnosis

MS | MS very unlikely | MS possible | Wide differential diagnosis

Action

Treat for MS | Reassure, reevaluate when appropriate | Close follow-up, individualized investigation | Focused work-up, extensive invasive testing may be warranted (Tables 5.10–5.15)

mitting after several weeks. Her examination reveals optic nerve dysfunction, corticospinal tract deficits, and sensory loss in the legs. Her brain magnetic resonance imaging (MRI) shows periventricular T2 hyperintensities consistent with demyelination; screening tests such as antinuclear antibodies (ANA) and serology for Lyme disease are negative. There is no evidence of peripheral nervous system involvement, other major systemic illness, or family history of neurological disease. In such a patient, MS is almost the only consideration, and diagnosis and treatment can be entered into with confidence and without the need for extensive testing or attention to a wide differential diagnosis.

Empirical support for this assertion comes from investigations such as that of the Rochester-Toronto MRI Study Group[250] in which *all* patients in whom there was stringent clinical *and* MRI evidence of MS at presentation had MS confirmed with prolonged follow-up and extensive testing; in other words, there are essentially no exceptions to the rule that MS is present if this diagnosis is achieved on the basis of *strict criteria* for *both* clinical and MRI findings. In the same study, however, it was found that there was a false-positive rate of diagnosis of 9% if less-stringent criteria were used, for example, if MRI findings that were only "probable" were accepted as indicative of MS.

The pattern of disease described (relapsing-remitting course with signs and symptoms highly suggestive of central nervous system [CNS] demyelination disseminated in time and space) is easily recognized by experienced clinicians. In such cases, many physicians will intuitively make the diagnosis of MS on the basis of bedside findings and informal application of laboratory tests such as MRI. Recently, however, evidence-based approaches have been applied to the diagnosis of MS, resulting in expert consensus statements and formal diagnostic criteria for this disease.

It is recommended that the clinician caring for MS patients be familiar with these criteria, and in many circumstances it may be helpful to have prepared checklists for laboratory workup, formal inclusionary criteria for MS, and atypical features casting doubt on the diagnosis of MS.

Investigation and Diagnostic Criteria, Typical Presentation of Multiple Sclerosis

In patients with typical features of MS (Table 5.1), extensive laboratory investigations are rarely warranted. A list of suggested screening investigations applicable to most patients is detailed in Table 5.2. Almost all patients in whom MS is suspected will have a head MRI performed, although this is not absolutely necessary for diagnosis (Table 5.3). Evoked potential studies, especially visual evoked responses (VER), may be useful in establishing dissemination of lesions to the optic nerves. Lumbar puncture for cerebrospinal fluid (CSF) analysis, almost universally obtained in the past, currently is performed in only approximately 10% of suspected MS cases, usually when clinical and MRI results are inconclusive. Classical CSF findings in MS include:

- Nonspecific findings such as moderate pleocytosis (10-20 cells/mm^3; however, >50 cells/mm^3 are unusual and may indicate an alternative diagnosis) and modest increase in total protein (50-70 mg/dL)
- More specific abnormalities, such as the presence of oligoclonal bands (discrete immunoglobulin densities on electrophoresis), and an increase in CSF immunoglobulin G (IgG) index or synthetic rate (increased intrathecal antibody production), indicative of an inflammatory response within the CNS.[233,278] The frequency of

TABLE 5.1 — INITIAL SIGNS AND SYMPTOMS OF MULTIPLE SCLEROSIS

Common
- Weakness in one or more limbs (40%)
- Monocular visual changes suggestive of optic neuritis (22%)
- Paresthesias (21%)
- Diplopia (12%)

Less Common (≤5%)
- Vertigo
- Micturation or bowel disturbance
- Lhermitte sign (electriclike shocks into spine or limbs with neck flexion)
- Trigeminal neuralgia
- Paroxysmal symptoms
- Dysarthria
- Ataxia

Uncommon (at onset)
- Pain
- Sexual dysfunction
- Cognitive dysfunction
- Movement disorder

Frequencies given are approximate and depend on population under study; 30% to 55% of patients are polysymptomatic at onset.

References 179, 231, and 278.

characteristic CSF findings in MS, such as oligoclonal bands or elevated IgG index, varies from approximately 40% to 50% in early, suspected cases to 85% to 95% in later, clinically definite cases. Thus at first presentation, a characteristic CSF pattern may support the diagnosis of MS, although a normal CSF does not rule it out. By contrast, in a patient with long-standing presumed MS, a normal CSF analysis indicates that this diagnosis should be entertained cautiously. It is also important to recall that CSF

TABLE 5.2 — SUGGESTED WORKUP FOR SUSPECTED MULTIPLE SCLEROSIS

Screening (all patients)
- History, neurological examination
- Brain magnetic resonance imaging (MRI)
- Routine blood counts, chemistries, urinalysis
- Lyme serology (ELISA) screen in endemic areas
- Antinuclear antibody (ANA)
- Rapid plasma reagin (RPR) or other serology for syphilis
- Vitamin B_{12} level
- Thyroid function tests

Secondary (if indicated clinically)
- Examination of cerebrospinal fluid (cell count, immunoglobulin G [IgG] index, oligoclonal bands)
- Evoked potentials (eg, visual evoked responses [VER])
- Lyme Western blot, Lyme cerebrospinal fluid (CSF) index (for strong suspicion of Lyme disease or positive screening tests)
- SS-A, SS-B antibodies (suspected Sjögren syndrome)
- Erythrocyte sedimentaion rate (ESR), antineutrophil cytoplasmic antibody (ANCA), anticardiolipin antibodies (suspected vasculitis or cerebrovascular disease)
- MRI of spinal cord (prominent cord signs or if head MRI is unexpectedly normal)
- Other tests as indicated in differential diagnosis (Tables 5.10 through 5.15)

Purists might argue that universal application of this screening panel is not strictly cost-effective, eg, in terms of the resources required to identify one case of neurosyphilis in the population tested. Also, in persons suspected of MS but otherwise normal, most positive determinations obtained will be false-positives. Nevertheless, the utility of the proposed workup from a clinical perspective is to "cast a wide net," ie, to maintain a high sensitivity or level of suspicion for conditions that might mimic MS and thus require a different treatment. Obviously, in terms of both performing and interpreting the workup, clinical judgment and critical use of tests are mandatory, and the investigations pursued must be tailored to each patient's individual presentation.

Adapted from References 69 and 83.

oligoclonal bands (and probably increased IgG synthesis) are common in other inflammatory CNS diseases and occasionally are found in noninflammatory neurological diseases[278]; thus positive CSF results, like positive MRI results, may be nonspecific.

In 2001, an international panel of experts chaired by Professor WI McDonald, reviewed and updated existing formal diagnostic criteria for MS.[234] The committee took into account new developments such as MRI and other paraclinical tests, while retaining the core concept of MS derived from Charcot[249] and used to define this disease for over a century, namely, the dissemination of clinical attacks and demyelinating lesions in time and space. The pragmatic, evidence-based recommendations of this committee are likely to be widely applied, both in clinical practice and in research. Essentially, the McDonald Committee indicates that the diagnosis of MS may be achieved by the following formula:

$$MS = DIS + DIT + NBE$$

Where:

DIS = lesions suggestive of MS, established by clinical or laboratory evidence and *disseminated in space*, ie, plaques of CNS demyelination

DIT = attacks suggestive of MS, established by objective clinical evaluation, *disseminated in time*, ie, recurrent episodes consistent with CNS demyelination

NBE = *No better explanation*, ie, clinical findings are unlikely to be caused by a condition other than MS

In order to apply the recommended criteria, the McDonald Committee indicated five clinical presentations or situations in which the diagnosis of MS is usually considered (Table 5.4). Operationally, in each

TABLE 5.3 — DIAGNOSTIC CRITERIA FOR MS, McDONALD COMMITTEE[1]

	Clinical Evidence at Presentation				Additional Clinical or Paraclinical Evidence *(italics)*[2] Required for MS Diagnosis	
	Clinical Setting/Condition	Attacks[3]	Lesions[4]	Criteria Proven[5]	DIS[6]	DIT[6]
1	Definite MS on clinical grounds	≥ 2	≥ 2	DIS, DIT	Already proven[7]	Already proven[7]
2	Localized disease	≥ 2	1	DIT only	2.1: Stringent MRI DIS or MRI and positive CSF or further clinical attack implicating a second site	Already proven
3	Multifocal attack	1	≥ 2	DIS only	Already proven	3.1: MRI DIT or second attack
4	Monosymptomatic demyelination (CIS)	1	1	Neither	4.1: Stringent MRI DIS or MRI and positive CSF	4.2: MRI DIT or second attack
5	Primary progressive disease	Course is insidious, with steady progression of clinical deficits			5.1: DIS by MRI in combinations with VER[8], and 5.3: Positive CSF	5.2: MRI DIT; or continued progression for 1 year

Abbreviations: CIS, clinically isolated syndrome; CSF, cerebrospinal fluid; DIS, disseminated in space; DIT, disseminated in time; MS, multiple sclerosis; MRI, magnetic resonance imaging; VER, visual evoked response.

1. Adapted and summarized from Reference 234. In some cases, terminological changes have been made for clarity of presentation. See the original report for detailed explanations.

2. Additional requirements for diagnosis. In clinical setting or condition #1, no further information is needed; in condition #2, evidence of DIS (2.1) is needed; in condition #3, evidence of DIT (3.1) is needed; in condition # 4, evidence for both DIS (4.1) and DIT (4.2) is needed; and in condition # 5, evidence for DIS (5.1), DIT (5.2), and positive CSF (5.3) is needed.

3. An attack (exacerbation, relapse) is defined as a clinical event, lasting 24 hours, suggestive of MS, and not consisting of worsening which are 1) observed directly or 2) based on historical report (eg, visual blurring), provided there are observed signs (eg, objective evidence of optic nerve dysfunction) compatible with the symptoms. To be considered a separate, second event, a further attack must start at least 30 days after the onset of the prior attack.

4. Lesions, suggestive of MS, revealed by clinical signs

5. Proof that MS is DIS or DIT, based on history and examination. In all cases, there should be no better explanation, ie, no evidence that a disease other than MS is likely to account for the patient's findings.

6. See Tables 5.8 and 5.9 for paraclinical, or laboratory, evidence that may be accepted in support of establishing DIS, DIT, and MS diagnosis. The distinction between "stringent MRI criteria" and "MRI and positive CSF" is explained in Table 5.8.

7. Additional studies are desirable (eg, MRI), even though MS is proven on clinical grounds. If performed, paraclinical tests are expected to be consistent with MS; if, unexpectedly, results are not supportive of MS, the diagnosis should be entertained with caution and reassessment considered.

8. Valid evidence for DIS in primary-progressive disease is different from evidence for DIS in relapsing-remitting disease, as explained in Table 5.8.

TABLE 5.4 — NARRATIVE EXPLANATION AND EXAMPLES: MCDONALD COMMITTEE CRITERIA FOR FIVE CLINICAL PRESENTATIONS

Definite Multiple Sclerosis on Clinical Grounds
(≥ 2 attacks, ≥ 2 lesions)

Example: First attack of optic neuritis, second attack with diplopia, clinical evidence of optic nerve and brain stem dysfunction, no better explanation or atypical features. The diagnosis of multiple sclerosis (MS) is established (disseminated in space [DIS], disseminated in time [DIT], no better explanation [NBE]), and no further workup is required. Nonetheless, as indicated in Table 5.3, paraclinical tests are usually performed and are expected to be confirmatory of MS

Localized Disease (≥ 2 attacks, 1 lesion)

Example: Two attacks of brain stem dysfunction, abnormal signs limited to brain stem. With this presentation, it is possible the patient's disease could represent a localized brain stem process such as a vascular malformation mimicking MS. Thus dissemination (2.1) of pathology throughout the central nervous system (CNS) in a manner typical of MS is required for diagnosis. This requirement is met by either stringent MRI criteria for DIS, ≥ 2 MRI lesions consistent with MS plus positive cerebrospinal fluid (CSF), or by a second attack implicating another site. The criteria for "positive CSF" are CSF-specific oligoclonal bands or elevated CSF immunoglobulin G (IgG) index

Multifocal Attack (1 attack, ≥ 2 lesions)

Example: Acute attack with evidence of widespread involvement of optic nerve, cerebellum, and spinal cord; this could represent an inherently monophasic disease such as acute disseminated encephalomyelitis following a viral illness. Thus for a diagnosis of MS, additional data are required to establish DIT (3.1), either by stringent MRI criteria or a second clinical attack

Monosymptomatic Attack (CIS) (1 attack, 1 lesion)

Example: Single attack with symptoms and signs limited to one area of spinal cord. This illness could represent spinal cord pathology such as transverse myelitis, without recurrent, widespread demyelination characteristic of MS. Thus additional data required for MS include both (4.1) DIS established by stringent MRI criteria or ≥ 2 MRI lesions plus positive CSF and (4.2) DIT established by either MRI criteria or a second attack

Primary-Progressive Disease
(insidious progression of deficits)

Example: A myelopathy presenting in middle age, with continuous worsening and no punctuated events. This illness could represent a compressive myelopathy due to localized disease such as a tumor or disk protrusion. Here, for a diagnosis of MS, all three additional criteria must be met: (5.1) DIS by MRI in combination with visual evoked responses (VER) (Table 5.9), (5.2) DIT by MRI criteria or clinical progression for a year, and (5.3) a positive CSF, indicating inflammation and therefore supporting MS specificity

5

instance, the clinician is prompted or asked whether sufficient clinical information exists to make the diagnosis of MS by the traditional formula above. If such information is not present, the criteria indicate what additional clinical or paraclinical data are required for diagnosis. After application of the criteria, there are three possible outcomes:

- MS (criteria are met; diagnosis is established)
- Possible MS (at risk for MS, but diagnostic evaluation equivocal at present)
- Not MS (criteria not met, current evaluation unequivocally negative).

A crucial component of the McDonald Committee recommendations is that there be no better explanation (NBE) for the patient's symptoms and signs. Logically, the NBE provision is circular; however, from a clinical perspective, this rule is very useful and indicates that a diagnosis of MS requires the critical judgment of an experienced clinician, especially as to whether another condition is likely to be present. Accordingly, the McDonald Committee indicates that "the diagnosis of MS remains a partly subjective and partly objective process."[234] In this regard, sets of features that cast doubt on the diagnosis of MS also have been proposed (Tables 5.5, 5.6, and 5.7). These criteria have been called red flags, or more properly yellow flags, since their presence, while not absolutely excluding MS, at least indicates that MS should be

---

TABLE 5.5 — NEUROLOGICAL RED FLAGS OR CAUTIONARY CRITERIA FOR MS*

- Absence of eye findings (optic nerve or oculomotor)
- Absence of clinical remission (more worrisome in a young patient)
- Localized disease (posterior fossa, craniocervical junction, spinal cord)
- Absence of sensory findings or absence of bladder involvement (since either or both are so common in most cases of established multiple sclerosis [MS])
- Absence of abnormalities on examination of cerebrospinal fluid or cranial magnetic resonance imaging (MRI) scan

Criteria do not exclude MS, since patients may present with a pure myelopathy or have a primarily progressive course (10%). The criteria have been modified to include neuroimaging; in the rare cases of MS in which cranial MRI is normal or almost normal, MRI imaging of the spinal cord usually provides evidence of demyelination.

* These criteria do not absolutely rule out MS. The red flags only indicate atypicality and doubt with regard to this diagnosis, thus indicating the need for caution and particularly careful evaluation.

Adapted from Reference 320.

TABLE 5.6 — GENETIC RED FLAGS OR CAUTIONARY CRITERIA FOR MS*

- Family history of MS (≥1 first-degree relatives)
- Early age at onset of MS (less than 15 years)
- Presence of unexplained non-CNS disease (eg, unexplained anemia, major dermatologic lesions, cardiomyopathy, organomegaly, proteinuria, metabolic acidosis, etc)

Abbreviations: MS, multiple sclerosis; CNS, central nervous system.

* These criteria do not absolutely rule out MS. The red flags only indicate atypicality and doubt with regard to this diagnosis, thus indicating the need for caution and particularly careful evaluation.

Adapted from: Reference 255.

accepted cautiously and that reevaluation of the patient is warranted.

As indicated, the McDonald Committee criteria validate the traditional diagnostic approach to MS based on clinical dissemination in space and time. However, the criteria also incorporate paraclinical evidence such as MRI, CSF results, and VER in instances where purely clinical data are insufficient for diagnosis, such as first attacks or clinically isolated syndromes (CIS) presentations. In this regard, the MRI findings supportive of a diagnosis of MS (Tables 5.8 and 5.9) may strike some as complex or unwieldy in their application; however, the indicated MRI findings have the advantage of having been carefully selected on the basis of empirical studies showing that they are reliably associated with MS.

Especially in intermediate cases, ie, when the MRI is not either floridly abnormal or absolutely normal, the use of such explicit, evidence-based criteria represents an advance over a vague or intuitive approach to ambiguous paraclinical data. Also, it should be

TABLE 5.7 — PSYCHIATRIC RED FLAGS OR CAUTIONARY CRITERIA FOR MS*

- Marked disproportion of symptoms relative to objective neurological signs
- Excessive emotional investment in being diagnosed with multiple sclerosis (MS), especially when this diagnosis appears tenuous or very unlikely by objective neurological assessment; abnormal, fearful response to the good news that MS is not present or is unlikely
- Prior history dominated by major psychiatric disease
- Unrelenting negative attitude, not explained by clinical depression, concerning prognosis, return of any function, or the possibility of coping with symptoms or life satisfactorily
- Tendency to confrontation, distrust of medical profession or scientific findings, politicalization of disease, a sense of victimization, nonreceptivity to psychotherapy or consideration of psychological factors

Psychiatric red flags are useful but must be applied with great caution. MS has presented as a psychotic illness, though often, neurological findings are evident at onset or shortly thereafter; also, minor psychiatric disturbance is common in the general population and may be present in many patients who subsequently develop MS. It is essential to distinguish between 1) primary psychiatric disease mimicking MS and 2) secondary psychiatric dysfunction in a person with MS due to brain lesions, psychosocial stress, or frustration with delayed diagnosis. It is the allover pattern, rather than one or two criteria, with the presence or absence of objective neurological findings, that is important in application of these criteria.

* These criteria do not absolutely rule out MS. The red flags only indicate atypicality and doubt with regard to this diagnosis, thus indicating the need for caution and particularly careful evaluation.

Adapted from References 244, 281, and author's experience.

TABLE 5.8 — MAGNETIC RESONANCE IMAGING CRITERIA FOR DISSEMINATION IN SPACE

Stringent MRI Criteria*

At least three of the following four criteria must be met:
- One gadolinium-enhancing lesion or nine T2-intense lesions
- $\geq$1 Infratentorial lesion (brain stem, cerebellum)
- $\geq$1 Juxtacortical lesion (U fibers, subcortical cerebral)
- $\geq$3 Periventricular lesion (abutting surface of lateral ventricle)

(Lesions are usually $\geq$3 mm in cross section. One spinal cord lesion can be substituted for one brain lesion.)

MRI Plus CSF Criteria[†]

Both of the following criteria must be met:
- $\geq$2 Lesions consistent with MS (ie, features above)
- CSF showing oligoclonal banding or increased IgG index

Abbreviations: CSF, cerebrospinal fluid; IgG, immunoglobulin G; MRI, magnetic resonance imaging; MS, multiple sclerosis.

In the case of progressive disease, clinical presentation #5 in Table 5.3, a variety of MRI findings are each accepted as evidence of DIS, including: 1) 9–T2-intense lesions or 2) 2 separate spinal cord lesions or 3) 4-8 brain lesions and 1 spinal cord lesion or 4) positive VER and 4-8 brain lesions or 5) positive VER with <4 lesions but 1 spinal cord lesion. Positive VER is defined by delayed but well-preserved waveforms consistent with MS. In all cases, it is assumed for valid application of the criteria that MRI, CSF, and VER analyses are performed reliably with careful controls and that abnormalities found are consistent with MS. The original study[234] should be consulted for details and explanations.

* Stringent MRI criteria (author's terminology) in which MRI evidence, based on studies by Barkhof et al[22] and Tintore et al,[378] are of high sensitivity and specificity for MS and thus stand alone.
† MRI evidence that is less compelling until supplemented by positive CSF data, presumably providing increased specificity to the MRI evidence.

Reference 234.

TABLE 5.9 — MAGNETIC RESONANCE IMAGING CRITERIA FOR DISSEMINATION IN TIME

Two circumstances are considered with regard to the timing of MRI relative to the presenting clinical event:

- If the first MRI is performed 3 months after the clinical event (MRI "delayed" in time), one of the two below must be found:
  - ≥ 1 Gadolinium-enhancing lesion, not at the site implicated in the original attack; or
  - If there is no gadolinium-enhancing lesion on this scan, a follow-up MRI should be performed 3 months later, and criteria are met if the follow-up scan shows a new T2 intense lesion or a gadolinium-enhancing lesion
- If the first MRI is performed <3 months after the clinical event (MRI done acutely), then a second MRI done 3 months after the attack provides evidence for DIT if one of the two criteria below are met:
  - A new gadolinium-enhancing lesion is observed (ie, present on the second scan but not present on the first scan); or
  - If criteria above is not met, and further (later) MRI studies are performed, these must show either new T2-intense lesions or gadolinium-enhancing lesions

Abbreviations: DIT, dissemination in time; MRI, magnetic resonance imaging; MS, multiple sclerosis.

The McDonald Committee[234] requires that MRI lesions are suggestive of MS. Thus, for examples, neither punctate T2 lesions nor a large gadolinium-enhancing lesion with mass effect is typical of MS and could not be used as MRI support in the criteria above.

---

pointed out that in all cases, the McDonald Committee's approach is to retain or begin with the core clinical concept of MS based on neurological findings typical of MS; while paraclinical evidence may be used to supplement or extend clinical evidence, sensitive but nonspecific tests such as MRI cannot be used in the absence of clinical evidence (MS diagnosis by MRI alone is not sanctioned). For example, CIS patients not meeting the clinical plus paraclinical criteria for MS (Table 5.3) remain patients with an isolated syndrome according to the McDonald Committee; technically, the *diagnosis* in these patients and the optimal *treatment* for these patients are different issues (see discussion of CHAMPS and ETOMS studies in Chapter 6, *Disease-Modifying Treatment*). In essence, the McDonald Committee avoids the extremes of inflexibly relying on either clinical or paraclinical diagnostic evidence to the exclusion of the other. Instead, the established, validated approach to MS diagnosis—clinical dissemination in time and space—is extended by evidence-based application of paraclinical testing.

After evaluating a patient suspected of having MS, a valuable clinical exercise is to use a prepared, printed list of inclusionary (eg, McDonald Committee, Table 5.3) and exclusionary (ie, red flags, Tables 5.5, 5.6, and 5.7) criteria. If all of the inclusionary criteria are met and none of the red flags are present, MS is very likely; if not, caution and further investigation are necessary. The consideration of atypical patients follows.

Group II: Atypical Multiple Sclerosis Presentation With Normal or Equivocal Neurological Findings

With regard to all patients suspected of having MS, the most important consideration is careful attention to a thorough history and detailed neurological examination. In group II patients, typical findings of MS (Table 5.1) are absent and full assessment reveals few or no symptoms or signs indicative of neurological dysfunction.

In this context, it has been suggested that MS be considered in the differential diagnosis of unexplained fatigue, minor sensory symptomatology, or subtle psychological change; nevertheless, in the absence of characteristic symptoms or objective signs, such patients *almost never* are found to have MS after extensive workup and prolonged observation. Specifically, conditions such as somatization disorder, chronic fatigue syndrome, chronic seronegative Lyme encephalopathy, fibromyalgia, panic disorder, benign paresthesias, and the like usually can be easily differentiated from MS by the absence of objective abnormalities on careful neurological examination.

Concern about MS in these settings is rarely warranted since MS is a chronic, progressive CNS disease that eventually *almost always* results in significant, obvious neurological dysfunction. In fact, apart from a thorough history and physical examination, extensive investigation of patients without characteristic symptoms or signs of neurological disease should generally be discouraged, since such adventures may only reveal false-positive, nonspecific findings or unproductively increase patient anxiety about a condition they do not have. Physician fears regarding legal liability for delayed diagnosis are best addressed by careful clinical assessment, close follow-up, communication with the patient, and documentation of a reasonable approach in the medical record, rather than inappropriate and excessive testing.

Patients with benign neurological presentations should be reassured, and primary, underlying psychological or medical issues addressed directly. At times, it may be useful to point out that minor symptoms such as fleeting sensory changes or nonspecific dizziness often are due to transient infections or metabolic imbalances that we do not fully understand but that usually do not cause serious or lasting disability.

In the *exceptional* case that remains doubtful or intractable despite the approach suggested above, periodic reassessment and paraclinical investigations may be appropriate for reassurance and to monitor the patient for the unexpected but possible development of objective neurological findings. In patients in whom MRI studies are performed, physicians should be aware that normal results provide very strong evidence against a diagnosis of MS. For example, in the large study by Thorpe and colleagues,[376] no patient with suspected MS (symptom duration 6 months to 18 years) in whom head *and* spinal MRIs were normal or near-normal was found to have MS. Also, minor and occasionally florid head MRI abnormalities may be noted in patients with migraine, tension headaches, psychiatric disease, normal aging, and other benign conditions,[20,91,188] thus indicating the need for caution when white matter lesions are identified in the absence of a relevant clinical correlate. In patients without evidence of significant neurological abnormalities, but in whom there is clear evidence of major psychological dysfunction, referral to a mental health specialist may be helpful (see Revealing the Diagnosis in Chapter 8, *Prognosis and Management*).

Group III: Atypical Multiple Sclerosis Presentation With Minor but Definite Neurological Findings

Group III patients, like group II patients, do not satisfy all diagnostic criteria for MS (Table 5.3); however, in contrast to group II patients, group III patients have subtle but definite symptoms or signs highly suggestive of MS or a related neurological disease. Terms such as "suggestive, possible, or probable" have been applied to these patients, and they may represent 30% to 40% of the population in which MS is an initial consideration; thus the diagnosis for group III patients is tentative, occupying an intermediate position between that of definite MS (group I) and definite non-MS (group II). For example, a patient may describe a previous attack of painful monocular visual impairment with recovery in several weeks, a story characteristic of optic neuritis; however, this patient may only have minor neurological abnormalities, eg, slight pallor of the optic nerve head on funduscopy or subjective diminution of color vision. Another patient may relate recurrent clumsiness or heaviness of the legs but have a normal neurological examination, apart from "soft" findings such as brisk stretch reflexes or an equivocal toe sign on plantar stimulation. Formally, group III patients meet some, but not all, inclusionary diagnostic criteria for MS. Also, in such patients, MRI findings often are equivocal at presentation; ie, MRI often is abnormal but does not demonstrate findings with high sensitivity and specificity for MS (Table 5.8).

Unlike group II patients in whom objective neurological dysfunction and, therefore, CNS disease is very improbable, group III patients demonstrate neurological findings that are definite but not at present specifically indicative of MS or any other neurological condition. Thus group III patients are heterogenous and diagnosistically challenging. Many of these patients will eventually be found to have unequivocal MS, while others will be found to have another serious neurological or systemic disease. Some will be found to be suffering from a relatively benign condition such as complicated migraine, low-grade cervical spondylosis, a mild postinfectious syndrome, or isolated, almost inapparent demyelination. In exceptional patients, no definite diagnosis or severe disability will be established after prolonged follow-up, extensive investigation, and careful reinvestigation. Empirically, a prospective study[133] of patients in which MS seemed *probable* on initial clinical evaluation found that MRI allowed a definite diagnosis of MS to be made in 50% of cases and a definite diagnosis of non-MS to be made in 10% of cases; in subjects in whom the clinical impression was *possible* MS, MRI assessment resulted in a diagnosis of MS in 5% of cases and non-MS in 25% of cases. It is evident from these results that even after a thorough workup, the diagnosis remains in doubt in a substantial portion of group III patients. Giang and associates[133] also found that CSF and evoked potential analysis resulted in very few possible-probable patients being reclassified as definite MS or non-MS; ie, the yield or additional value of these tests was very low at initial presentation. In all cases, obviously, the gold standard for diagnosis remains the subsequent clinical course of the patient.

How then should atypical cases suggestive of but not currently reaching the diagnostic threshold for definite MS be worked up? First, regular follow-up with careful neurological reassessment is essential in all cases. Second, a key question for patient and physician is the *extent to which intensive investigation is currently desirable.* For example, some patients have minimal clinical and MRI findings, suggesting a relatively good prognosis (see Chapter 8) and are comfortable with watchful waiting, reluctant to undergo procedures such as lumbar puncture, compliant with clinic visits, and tolerant of uncertainty. For such patients, continued observation and periodic reinvestigation (eg, clinical examination and MRI perhaps at yearly or more frequent intervals until diagnosis is clear) may be appropriate. At the other extreme are patients who have substantial clinical and MRI evidence of disease activity and are anxious to "get to the bottom of things," accepting of investigations, and intolerant of uncertainty. For such patients, investigations such as lumbar puncture, evoked potentials, secondary serologies, and the like should be performed and may indicate that MS is present or highly likely.

All patients should understand that an instant and infallible diagnosis is not always possible,[133] that sometimes all investigations will be inconclusive, and that in these circumstances a deferred opinion and reassessment are the best strategies. Almost all patients will respond positively to a sympathetic, honest explanation of diagnostic uncertainty, especially when it is coupled with a rational and directed plan for close follow-up. Finally, physicians should be aware of reports such as the CHAMPS[171] and ETOMS[71] studies, which have shown benefits associated with prompt treatment of patients with incipient or early MS; discussion of this topic is presented in Chapter 6.

Group IV: Atypical Multiple Sclerosis Presentation With Major Neurological Findings

A final group of atypical patients will have substantial neurological findings such as a hemiplegia, marked visual loss, dementia, ophthalmoplegia, progressive paraparesis, progressive ataxia, or other evidence of serious and unequivocal neurological disease. Often such patients will have an acute or fulminant presentation requiring emergency evaluation or hospitalization. Nonetheless, the initial neurological workup of such patients does not establish typical MS and may even suggest the substantial possibility of another disease; thus the NBE criterion of the McDonald Committee[234] is not met.

In some series, group IV patients may represent 5% of the population of patients suspected of having MS. In many group IV patients, the correct diagnosis will be clear early in disease course; however, for those in which an obvious structural lesion or similar etiology is not immediately evident, a wide differential diagnosis exists, as indicated in Tables 5.10 through 5.15. Many of the conditions listed are quite rare, but it is sobering that each of the diseases indicated in Tables 5.10 through 5.15 has been misdiagnosed as MS, as documented in the cited case reports and reviews. It is also true on probabilistic grounds that in any given patient, an atypical presentation of MS is more likely than the occurrence of a very rare condition such as Eales disease or an adult-onset leukodystrophy. Nonetheless, for the patient who is suffering from an unusual disease mimicking MS, especially one that is treatable, such as a metabolic defect of B_{12} metabolism or Sjogren's syndrome or Hashimoto encephalopathy, the probability of misdiagnosis and mistreatment is 100% when their malady is not *considered* in the differential diagnosis. The lists in Tables 5.10 through 5.15 have been prepared as an overview in this regard; particular emphasis has been placed on features or clinical patterns that should raise the suspicion of a given condition and initial measures that should be undertaken to screen for each disease. In view of the importance of MRI in MS diagnosis, specific neuroimaging features have been indicated, when known, for each condition.

How, then, should patients in group IV be approached? Initially, a patient's clinical and MRI findings usually are indicative of a specific subgroup, for example:

- *Immunological* (Table 5.10) (acute leukoencephalopathy presentation, CSF pleocytosis, evidence of systemic autoimmunity, involvement of blood vessels in eye or other site)
- *Infectious* (Table 5.11) (exposure, serology, fever, characteristic skin lesions)
- *Degenerative* (Table 5.12) (strong family history, abnormal blood chemistries, diffuse white matter disease seen on MRI)
- *Oncological* (Table 5.13) (known or suspected neoplasm, relentless course)
- *Spinal cord disease* (Table 5.14) (progressive myelopathy, with few signs of involvement "above the neck"; may overlap with categories above)
- *Toxic/miscellaneous* (Table 5.15) (history of industrial, medical, or personal exposure)

TABLE 5.10A — DIFFERENTIAL DIAGNOSIS OF MS: IMMUNOLOGICAL—MS VARIANTS

Disease[1]	Cardinal Features[2]	Screening[3]	MRI[4]	Comments[5]
Monosymptomatic demyelination (CIS)	A single attack (eg. optic neuritis or brain stem dysfunction) suggestive of demyelination	As per MS (Table 5.2)	H: a single lesion or several lesions suggestive of MS; MRI of CIS discussed in Chapter 4	Management discussed in Chapter 6; may represent "incipient" or pathological MS
Transverse myelitis	Acute attack with evidence of spinal dysfunction below a defined level, often with symmetrical signs ("complete myelitis"), rather than assymmetry of typical myelopathy due to MS	As per MS; spinal MRI and CSF examination essential; presence of oligoclonal bands favors MS; search for systemic disease or viral CSF infection, as transverse myelitis is often a diagnosis of exclusion	M: spinal MRI often shows extensive signal change; brain MRI may be normal in classic transverse myelitis; if brain MRI shows many demyelinating lesions, MS is more likely (see Chapter 4, CIS discussion)	Relationship of transverse myelitis to MS is complex[6,174], although transverse myelitis typically is monophasic, relapsing forms have been described[379]
Balo concentric sclerosis	MS variant with atypical lesions showing alternating bands or lamelli of demyelination and preserved WM	As per MS; autopsy reveals characteristic lesions	M: concentric WM lesions may be mixed with typical MS lesions[199]	Treatment uncertain; possibly steroids; immunosuppression, plasma exchange[217]
Myelinoclastic diffuse sclerosis (Schilder disease)	Bilateral hemispheric demyelination, onset usually in childhood; aphasia, dementia, seizures, increased intracranial pressure	As per MS; rule out leukodystrophies, especially adrenoleukodystrophy	M: large confluent areas of T2I in WM	Classification, terminology controversial[217]

Tumefactive MS	Large focus of demyelination, often with mass effect and edema, resembling a brain tumor; patient may present with headache, focal signs, seizures	MRI; MRS; may require brain biopsy, although misdiagnosis is possible, even histologically[287]	M: large, tumorlike lesion, with or without other lesions characteristic of MS; a pattern of open-ring enhancement at the border of the lesion may favor demyelination vs primary tumor[112,227]	Subsequent clinical course variable, sometimes mono-phasic; biopsy may be hyper-cellular with tumor differen-tiation difficult, but presence of macrophages and myelin loss with relative preserva-tion of axons should lead to correct diagnosis[217]
Marburg disease	Fulminant, acute demyelina-tion of cerebrum and/or brain stem	As per MS	M: few MRI reports; pathol-ogy suggestions extensive lesions with evidence of tissue loss will be present	Often relentless progres-sion to death in <12 mo; pathology shows necrosis and axonal destruction; treat with steroids, immuno-suppression, or plasma ex-change[217]
Devic disease (neuromyelitis optica)	Severe monophasic or relaps-ing demyelination affecting optic nerves and spinal cord	As per MS; may be associated with SLE	M: dramatic changes in cervi-cal cord MRI with swelling and edema sometimes mimicking tumor; brain MRI may or may not show periventricular demye-lination[223]	Fulminant demyelination with necrosis; CSF (often neutrophils are present and oligoclonal bands are ab-sent) and lack of HLA association suggest this is a distinct MS variant[408]

Continued

Disease[1]	Cardinal Features[2]	Screening[3]	MRI[4]	Comments[5]
Chronic inflammatory demyelinating polyneuropathy	Progressive relapsing demyelination predominantly affecting the PNS, but sometimes associated with CNS demyelination[375]	Electrodiagnostic studies, CSF with high albumin and low cells	M: T2I have been described, but usually are not as widespread as lesions in classic MS[115]	Definitive test is nerve biopsy; occasionally MS patients may have evidence of peripheral nerve abnormalities[393]
Acute disseminated encephalomeyelitis	Monophasic demyelination, often 1-2 weeks after infection or vaccination, often with altered level of consciousness	As per MS	H: often lesions appear to be of same age or stage of development; high lesion load; hyperacute form may be hemorrhagic or involve GM; GM or thalamic lesions may favor ADEM, and corpus callosum lesions may favor MS, but MRI may be identical in the two conditions[169,189,341]	More common in childhood, sometimes with explosive course[169]; prediction of MS development is difficult but in adults, preceding infection, brain stem involvement, high CSF albumin, and infratentorial lesions are more likely to be associated with final diagnosis of ADEM[341]
Bickerstaff brain stem encephalitis	Subacute inflammatory brain stem syndrome in a young adult, often after a prodrome of headache and malaise for weeks or months; ophthalmoplegia, ataxia, facial weakness, sensory symptoms, dysarthria, deafness; typically monophasic and with full recovery[130]	As per MS; CSF usually does not show oligoclonal bands and lymphocytic pleocytosis may be moderate or higher than typical MS	M: T2I diffusely through upper mesencephalon and thalamus[151,410]	Status of BBE uncertain (viral, postinfectious, first attack of MS); suspect in a young adult with fulminant brain stem syndrome and marked CSF pleocytosis

Abbreviations: ACE, angiotensin-converting enzyme; ACTH, adrenocorticotropic hormone; ADEM, acute disseminated encephalomyelitis; AIDS, acquired immunodeficiency syndrome; ALA, aminolevulinic acid; ALDP, adrenoleukodystrophy protein; ANA, antinuclear antibody; APBD, adult polyglusan body disease; APS, antiphospholipid antibody syndrome; aPTT, activated partial thromboplastin time; ATPase, adenosine triphosphatase; BBE, Bickerstaff brain stem encephalitis; BD, Binswanger disease; BSE, bovine spongiform encephalopathy; c-ANCA, cytoplasmic antineutrophilic cytoplasmic antibody; CADASIL, cerebral autosomal dominant arteriopathy with subcortical infarcts and leukoencephalopathy; CD, celiac disease; CD4 [cells], HIV helper cell count; CIS, clinically isolated syndromes; CJD, Creutzfeldt-Jakob disease; CNS, central nervous system; CPM, central pontine myelinolysis; CRV, cerebroretinal vasculopathy; CSC, central serous chorioretinopathy; CSF, cerebrospinal fluid; CT, computed tomography; dsDNA, double-stranded DNA; EEG, electro-encephalogram; ELISA, enzyme-linked immunosorbent assay; EMG, electromyogram; EMS, eosinophilia-myalgia syndrome; EPM, extrapontine myeli-nolysis; ESR, erythrocyte sedimentation rate; 5-FU, 5-fluorouracil; FLAIR, fluid attenuated inversion recovery; FTA-ABS, fluorescent treponemal anti-body absorpton [test]; GI, gastrointestinal; GM, gray matter; HCV, hepatitis C virus; HERNS, hereditary endotheliopathy, retinopathy, nephropathy, stroke; HHV, human herpes virus; HIV, human immunodeficiency virus; HLA, human leukocyte antigen; HSP, hereditary spastic paraparesis; HTLV-1, human T-cell lymphotropic virus, type 1; IgG, immunoglobulin G; IgM, immunoglobulin M; IV, intravenous; LA, leukoariosis; LHON, leber hereditary optic neur-opathy; MDMA ["ecstasy"], methylenedioxymethamphetamine; MELAS, mitochondrial encephalopathy with lactic acidosis and strokelike episodes; MERRF, myoclonic epilepsy with ragged red fibers; MHA-TP, microhemagglutination test for *Treponema pallidum*; MLD, metachromatic leukodystrophy; MNGIE, mitochondrial neurogastrointestinal encephalopathy; MRA, magnetic resonance angiography; MRI, magnetic resonance imaging; MRS, magnetic reso-nance spectometry; MS, multiple sclerosis; MTHRF, methylenetetrahydrofolate; MTR, magnetization transfer ratio; NARP, neuropathy, ataxia, retinitis pigmentosa; nvCJD, new variant Creutzfeldt-Jakob disease; OMIM, online Mendelian inheritance in man; OPCA, olivopontocerebellar atrophy; p-ANCA, perinuclear antineutrophilic cytoplasmic antibody; PBG, porphobilinogen; PCR, polymerase chain reaction; PML, progressive multifocal leukoencephal-opathy; PNS, peripheral nervous system; PrPSc, protease-resistant prion protein; PVL, periventricular leukomalacia; RBC, red blood [cell] count; RPR, rapid plasmin reagin [test]; SCAs, spinocerebellar ataxias; SLE, systemic lupus erythematosus; SS, Sjögrens syndrome; SSPE, subacute sclerosing panencephalitis; tRNA, transer ribonucleic acid; T2I, T2 hyperintensities (in WM unless otherwise stated); TTPA, triethylene thiophosphoramide; U [fi-bers], short association tracts connecting the adjacent gyri of the cerebrum; VDRL, Veneral Disease Research Laboratory [test for syphilis]; VER, visual evoked response; VLCFA, very long chain fatty acids; WBC, white blood [cell] count; WM, white matter.

Continued

5

Key: H, high probability that scan will be similar or identical to MS; M, middle probability of overlap with MS, usually some distinguishing features are present; L, low probability of overlap with MS, scans usually are very differentiating; U, unknown, few well-documented MRI reports in the literature.

General discussions of the relationship of MS to the variants above may be found in Lucchinetti,[217] Weinshenker,[402] and comprehensive MS reference texts.

1. Diseases that may realistically present with MS-like features and be included in the differential diagnosis. The emphasis has been placed on circumstances or reports in the literature in which diagnostic overlap has been noted. For example, typical SLE and MS usually are easily distinguished in the majority of cases. In Table 5.10B, however, the discussion has been focused on the minority of patients in whom SLE and MS have been found to cause diagnostic difficulty; in other words, the tables are biased toward instances in which diseases overlap, rather than typical, "classic" presentations in which differential diagnosis is not an issue.

2. Key or defining features that should alert the clinician to the possibility that a disease mimicking MS is present and assist with its recognition.

3. Screening or preliminary investigations that should be performed when the disease is suspected and that will assist with the decision to pursue definitive workup.

4. Given the essential role that brain MRI studies play in MS diagnosis, specific MRI (head study, unless stated otherwise) features of the disease under consideration are listed. In each case, the likelihood that MRI findings will overlap with those of MS are indicated. In some reports in which differential MRI diagnosis with MS has been specifically addressed, a citation is listed. In-depth discussion of MRI in the differential diagnosis of MS may be found in reference texts, Triulizi and Scotti,[385] and van der Knapp and Valk.[388]

5. Differentiating features and citations for in-depth discussion of the disease are indicated. Original sources should be consulted if an extensive or invasive workup is anticipated.

TABLE 5.10B — DIFFERENTIAL DIAGNOSIS OF MS: IMMUNOLOGICAL—INFLAMMATORY/RHEUMATOLOGICAL

Disease	Cardinal Features	Screening	MRI	Comments
Eale disease	Idiopathic retinalocclusive vasculopathy, sometimes with retinal hemorrhages; may cause visual blurring in young adults	Opthalmological examination; fluorescein angiogram; rare in North America, more common in Middle East; may be associated with tuberculosis	M: MS-like lesions and CSF findings have been reported[14,315]	May cause visual loss mimicking optic neuritis; neurological involvement includes internuclear opthalmoplegia, strokelike episodes, vestibuloauditory dysfunction, myelopathy, chronic encephalitis[18,394]
Bechet disease	Aphthous oral ulcerations, genital ulcers, uveitis, arthritis with predilection for Mediterranean, Middle East, Asian countries	CSF may show pleocytosis beyond the range of MS; biopsy of mucocutaneous lesions	M to H: WM changes identical to MS may be noted, although lesions of Bechet disease tend to be smaller and isolated; Bechet disease may prominently affect brain stem and deep GM; occasionally venous infarctions may occur[210,246,395]	May present with brain stem dysfunction, strokelike episodes, meningoencephalitis, intracranial hypertension, relapsing-remitting myelopathy[57,192]

Continued

5

Disease	Cardinal Features	Screening	MRI	Comments
Sarcoidosis	Multisystem disease with non-caseating granuloma; may mimic MS when optic nerve and/or spinal cord are involved	Serum ACE (low sensitivity); chest radiograph; gallium 67 lung scan; CSF ACE may be elevated; a minority of neurosarcoid patients have elevated CSF IgG or oligoclonal bands	M to H: WM changes may mimic MS; enhancement of meninges, hypothalamic lesions, lesions, or lesions at brain surface favors sarcoidosis[292,388]	Biopsy of skin, lung, lymph node, muscle, brain, or other site may be required to definitely establish sarcoidosis, particularly if systemic clinical findings are not typical[318]
Sjögrens syndrome (SS)	Autoimmune disease characterized by dry eyes, dry mouth, and other findings (arthritis, vasculitis, Raynaud phenomenon); MRI findings, relapsing-remitting course, excellent response to corticosteroids; neuropsychiatric symptoms may overlap MS[10]	Serology for SS-A (Ro), SS-B (La), rheumatoid factor; CSF may show oligoclonal bands and increased IgG synthesis	H: asymptomatic T2l in deep and subcortical WM are frequent in SS but of questionable clinical significance; corpus callosum lesions are frequent in MS but were not observed in a large series of SS patients[68]	Although controversial, most neurological and rheumatological authorities suggest that SS rarely has significant neurological manifestations[10,318]; auto-antibody screen and minor salivary gland biopsy if necessary should differentiate SS and MS. Skin lesions and peripheral neuropathy are common in SS and rare in MS

Systemic lupus erythematosus (SLE)	Multiorgan autoimmune disease; pathogenesis depends on autoantibodies, immune complexes, and vascular damage; may present with strokes, mental changes, myelopathy, optic nerve involvement, peripheral neuropathy, or other neurological manifestations	ANA, antibodies to dsDNA, presence of disease in many organs (renal, skin, musculoskeletal, pulmonary, hematologic); 60% show oligoclonal bands or IgG increase in CSF	H: WM changes similar to MS; additionally, peripheral WM lesions and strokelike lesions may be seen[188]	SLE features that may cause confusion include fluctuating course, involvement of optic nerve or spinal cord, similar CSF findings; also, about 30% of MS patients have modest ANA positivity; SLE depends on vasculopathy, MS on demyelination; differentiation can be difficult at times, but lack of systemic manifestations favors MS[228,318]
Eosinophilia-myalgia syndrome (EMS)	Myalgia, eosinophilia, systemic symptoms (liver, skin, lungs) with variable neurological manifestations (peripheral neuropathy, cognitive changes, muscle pain and weakness, diplopia), either idiopathic or after exposure to L-tryptophan	Complete blood count (≥1000 eosinophil/mm³); absence of infection or neoplasm	H: periventricular and deep WM T2[15,220]	Status of syndrome debated by rheumatologists[36]; CSF should not have typical MS-like findings

Abbreviations and Key: See Table 5.10A.

5

TABLE 5.10C — DIFFERENTIAL DIAGNOSIS OF MS: IMMUNOLOGICAL—VASCULAR

Disease	Features	Screening	MRI	Comments
Uveitis (or inflammatory ocular disease)	Inflammation of uvea, iris, or retina is reported in MS and in primary ocular or systemic diseases mimicking MS	Ophthalmologic examination, fluorescein angiography	H to L, depending on etiology: in some cases of uveitis associated with systemic diseases, MRI may closely mimic MS[44]	20% of MS patients have asymptomatic retinal vein sheathing; 2% of MS patients have symptomatic uveitis (eg, pars planitis); uveitis may be due to a primary systemic disease such as vasculitis, sarcoidosis, or infection[318,361]
Cogan syndrome	Interstitial keratitis associated with vertigo, tinnitus, hearing loss; at times with uveitis and CNS manifestations (vasculitis, encephalopathy, ataxia)	Prominent auditory loss, vestibular dysfunction; ophthalmological evaluation	M: T2I in WM reported,[56] although MRI is normal in other reports	Suspect in young patient with prominent ocular findings, including keratitis, with attacks resembling Menieres disease[82]
Susac syndrome	Microangiopathy of brain, retina, and cochlea	Ophthalmological evaluation, fluorescein angiography, audiology; CSF shows mild pleocytosis without IgG elevation or oligoclonal bands	M: WM changes similar to MS reported, though Susac may also involve GM	Diagnosis established by demonstrating angiopathy affecting small vessels in the three key organs[276,288]

Sneddon syndrome	Livedo reticularis, cerebro-vascular disease	Antiphospholipid antibodies, angiography, skin biopsy (relatively specific)	L: multiple small lesions consistent with strokes in WM and GM	Suspect in a young patient with recurrent strokelike attacks and lacy, network pattern of skin mottling in limbs and trunk[364,381]
Degos disease	Multisystem endothelial vasculopathy, with variable neurological symptoms, including paresthesias, weakness, monocular visual defects, changes in behavior or cognition, strokes, myelopathy, and neuropathy	Skin lesions that have a porcelain white center surrounded by a pink ring; antiphospholipid antibodies and immunoglobulin deposits have been described; CSF usually shows only increased protein, although oligoclonal bands have been noted in a few patients	M: shows strokes or non-specific focal abnormalities of WM or GM	Skin lesions are pathognomonic; stepwise progression of the illness occasionally has led to misdiagnosis of MS[318,366]
Vasculitis	Manifestations may be limited to CNS or associated with multiorgan involvement; see Rosenbaum[318] or Younger[415] for reviews of different types of vasculitis that affect the CNS	ESR, ANA, p-ANCA, c-ANCA, c-CSF, MRA; search for systemic manifestations of specific vasculitis or rematic disease	M: usually infarcts with prominent GM involvement; primary CNS vasculitis has been associated with T2I in periventricular and deep WM which has mimicked MS[187]	Unlike MS, vasculitis often presents with early cognitive and behavioral changes; usually angiography and brain biopsy are required if diagnosis is not established from systemic involvement[251]

Continued

105

Disease	Features	Screening	MRI	Comments
Antiphospholipid antibody syndrome (APS)	Recurrent venous or arterial occlusions; may present with subtle sensory or motor episodes; often manifest as a progressive myelopathy spinocerebellar, or neuromyelitis optica-type syndrome; may be idiopathic or associated with SLE or SS	IgG and IgM anticardiolipid antibodies, lupus anticoagulant tests (Russell viper venom time, kaolin clotting time); CSF shows oligoclonal bands in 15% of patients and cell count is usually normal	H: WM may show multifocal WM lesions, diffuse or confluent	APS favored by high titers of autoantibodies, headaches, seizures, strokelike attacks, systemic involvement (thrombosis, skin, arthritis, fetal loss, myocardial infarction)[47,87,182,328]
Central serous chorioretinopathy (CSC)	Recurrent, unilateral visual loss in young to middle-aged adults due to a serous detachment of the retina at the macula	Ophthalmological evaluation (usually, color vision is normal, afferent pupillary defect absent, fovea reflex lost); fluorescein angiography	L: CNS is not involved; apart from nonspecific or incidental findings, MRI is expected to be normal	CSC has been misdiagnosed as optic neuritis and MS when "soft" neurological signs are present[147,202]
Venous occlusive and cardioembolic disease	Recurrent attacks with focal deficits in young patient without obvious stroke risk factors	Tests for hypercoagulable state (deficiency of protein C, protein S, antithrombin III; activated protein C resistance, prothrombin gene mutation[55]; transesophageal echocardiography; prior personal or family history of venous occlusions	L: strokelike lesions usually do not resemble MS, unless involvement is subtle and primarily in WM	Historically, recurrent episodes with sudden onset should suggest atypical cerebrovascular disease

Migraine	Patient with characteristic migraine headaches and additional minor neurological symptoms or signs undergoes MRI scan and is found to have abnormalities	Uncomplicated migraine is not associated with definite, persisting neurological deficits	M: subtle WM lesions have been reported in children and adults with migraine, including accentuated perivascular spaces, small infarcts, and gliosis[91,335]	In difficult cases, CSF and evoked potential testing may be useful; MTR studies may differentiate MS and migraine[314]
Leukoariosis (LA), Binswanger disease (BD)	WM rarefacation defined radiologically (LA, punctate or patchy T2I in periventricular or deep cerebral WM) or clinically (BD, vascular leukoencephalopathy with dementia)	Screen for cerebrovascular risk factors, including age, hypertension, diabetes; neuropsychological assessment	M to H: lesions may be similar to MS; typically, in MS, WM U fibers are involved, but spared in LA-BD; in LA-BD, basal ganglia and GM may be involved but usually are not prominently involved in MS[167,388]	In difficult cases, differentiate by clinical setting, normal CSF[167,236]
Neuroretinitis (Leber Stellate retinitis)	Unilateral visual loss due to optic nerve capillary leak, often with subsequent macular star formation	Ophthalmological assessment, serology for syphilis, exposure to cat scratch, fluorescein angiography	L: expected to be normal	Neuroretinitis may mimic optic neuritis and in association with "soft" neurological signs lead to misdiagnosis of MS; neuroretinitis may be idiopathic or secondary to cat-scratch disease or syphilis; may be unilateral, bilateral-simultaneous, or bilateral-sequential; no increased MS risk[148,306]

Abbreviations and Key: See Table 5.10A.

5

TABLE 5.11 — DIFFERENTIAL DIAGNOSIS OF MULTIPLE SCLEROSIS: INFECTIOUS

Disease	Features	Screening	MRI	Comments
Progressive multifocal leukoencephalopathy (PML)	CNS infection by JC virus, usually in a patient with known immunodeficiency, relentless progression of deficits in cognition, language, vision; rarely, fluctuating case may mimic MS	Urine cytology, possibly PCR on urinary cells; CSF PCR 60%-100% sensitivity in compatible clinical setting[95]	M to H: T2I in WM, usually more confluent than MS, often contrast-enhancing, sometimes with mass effect[299]	Definitive diagnosis by brain biopsy, if required
Whipple disease	CNS infection by bacillus, most commonly causing dementia, eye movement abnormalities, myoclonus, rarely myelopathy, variable but steady progression	History of malabsorption; CSF PCR for specific bacillus[390]	M: variable with prominent atrophy and GM involvement; rarely T2I in WM reported[101,336]	Usually systemic manifestations (GI, joints) are present; if CSF screen does not establish diagnosis, small bowel biopsy and PCR definitive[13,224]
HTLV-1 myelopathy	Thoracic progressive myelopathy, rarely cerebral symptoms such as cognitive impairment	Risk factors for AIDS; origin or travel in Caribbean or Japan; serology for HTLV-1; CSF may show oligoclonal bands	M: spinal cord usually only shows atrophy, but brain may show small T2I in cerebral periventricular areas[205]	Positive serology favors HTLV-1; cranial nerve involvement, extensive brain and cervical MRI lesions, VER assymetry favors MS[319]
Lyme disease (neuroborreliosis)	Neurological complications (meningitis, neuropathy,	Endemic area and history of of exposure; prior headache,	M to H: T2I described, but usually not periventricular;	If serological screen is positive or equivocal, definitive

	encephalomyelitis) of infection by tick-borne by spirochete Borrelia burgdorferi	erythema migrans rash, arthritis; positive screening serology (eg, ELISA)	meningeal enhancement of basal ganglia involvement favors Lyme vs MS[117,307]	diagnosis by western blot and CSF lyme index[11,318,362]
Syphilis	Optic neuritis, vasculitis, myelopathy, chronic encephalopathy due to Treponema pallidum	Serology for RPR or VDRL (60%-98% sensitive); CSF for cells, protein, VDRL	M: Findings depend on stage of syphilis and may include infarction, nonspecific WM lesions, mass lesions (gumma), and meningeal enhancement[154]	Negative serology for specific Treponema determinants (FTA-ABS, MHA-TP) essentially rules out syphilis; use of CSF PCR, antibody indices advocated by some authorities[113,382]
HIV-1 leukoencephalopathy	HIV-1 infection usually causes typical AIDS dementia complex, but rarely HIV-1 can cause a more subtle, relapsing disease mimicking MS (optic neuritis, myelopathy, mental status changes)	Risk factors for exposure; HIV-1 serology; diminished CD4 cells	M: T2I in WM, often larger and more confluent than those of typical MS	HIV-1 leukoencephalopathy episodes often of sudden onset and limited recovery; CSF and evoked potentials may mimic MS[35,140]
New Variant Creutzfeldt-Jakob Disease (nvCJD)	Spongiform encephalopathy resembling classic CJD, but occurring in younger patients, often initially with psychiatric and sensory disturbances; due to infection with the BSE agent ("mad cow disease")	Clinical recognition; possibly biopsy of tonsil for PrPSc protein; all nvCJD patients are homozygous for methionine at codon 129 of the prion protein gene	L: normal or mild atrophy; rarely T2I reported in posterior cerebrum	Within several months of presentation, relentless progression and dementia should allow distinction from MS[305,316,397]; registry for CID cases: 216-368-0587 or www.cjdsurveillance.com

Continued

Disease	Features	Screening	MRI	Comments
Brucellosis	Rare in developed countries; associated with agricultural or animal exposure; clinical manifestations include depression, headache, PNS symptoms; optic neuritis, myelopathy, and "demyelinating syndromes" have been reported	Specific antibodies in serum and CSF	M: periventricular T2I have been reported	Brucellosis tends to involve many systems, including heart, eyes, lungs; often with fever and prominent meningoencephalitis with positive antibodies in CSF[4,412]
Subacute sclerosing panencephalitis (SSPE)	Chronic CNS infection by measles virus; onset usually in childhood but rarely in adolescents or adults; abnormal behavior, learning, myoclonus; usually progressive but sometimes relapsing-remitting; can follow natural measles or, more rarely, measles vaccine	Relative youth, prominent CSF oligioclonal bands directed against measles virus; EEG with paroxysmal bursting pattern	M: early in disease T2I in central cerebral WM; late in disease widespread, confluent lesions may spread to GM[388]	Eventually distinguished by relentless course, prominent dementia; definitive diagnosis by brain biopsy or CSF PCR[380]
Human Herpes Virus-6 (HHV-6)	Agent of exanthum subitum in infants, after which CNS latency may be established; reactivation implicated in a subacute MS-like syndrome[58] or myelopathy[221]	Serology for HHV-6	H: available pathology and CT reports indicate appearances could closely resemble MRI in MS	Etiologic relationship to MS currently the subject of intensive research

Hepatitis C virus (HCV)	Neurological complications of HCV most commonly involve the PNS; however, CNS syndromes including encephalopathy and optic neuropathy have been reported[372]	Serum antibodies and PCR for HCV; most patients are positive for serum cryoglobulins	H: diffuse or patchy areas of T2I in periventricular and deep WM; punctate areas of enhancement	Suspect in setting of IV drug abuse, transfusions, active liver disease; CNS manifestations often associated with simultaneous PNS diseases, such as polyneuropathy
Mycoplasma	Usually presents with an atypical pneumonia (2-3 weeks fever, malaise, headache, pronounced cough); neurological complications are rare but encephalitis, meningitis, transverse myelitis, brain stem involvement, cranial neuropathies, and PNS syndromes have been documented	Cold agglutinins in serum; specific antibodies in serum (acute and convalescent) and CSF; marked CSF pleocytosis (>100 cells) outside of typical MS range	H: confluent or punctate T2I in WM have been reported, usually with positive enhancement acutely[48]	Differentiate by fever, specific antibodies, systemic symptoms, monophasic course[30,240]

Abbreviations and Key: See Table 5.10A.

5

111

TABLE 5.12A — DIFFERENTIAL DIAGNOSIS OF MS: DEGENERATIVE—METABOLIC

Disease	Features	Screening	MRI	Comments
Central pontine (CPM) or extrapontine (EPM) myelinolysis	Demyelination of pons or other sites, often after rapid correction of hyponatremia in the setting of alcoholism or acute disease, usually severely ill (mental confusion, coma, bulbar syndrome, tetrapareses); rarely mild clinical manifestations	History of hyponatremia or other fluid or electrolyte disturbances	L to M: classic CPM has solitary pontine lesion, sometimes with 1-2 week delay in appearance; occasionally T2I WM change will be extensive, multiple, or confluent[204,388]	Clinical confusion with MS has occurred in younger patients with subtle CPM or EPM and occult risk factors (eg, eating disorder); clinical course and CSF should be differentiating
Hashimoto encephalopathy	Subacute, relapsing-remitting encephalopathy (confusion, myoclonus, strokelike episodes, depressed consciousness) associated with autoimmune thyroid disease	High titers of antithyroglobulin, antimicrosomal antibodies (note: routine thyroid function tests may be normal); diffusely abnormal EEG, high CSF protein without pleocytosis	L to M: may be normal, but transient, focal, and diffuse T2I in WM have been reported[40]	Suspect Hashimoto disease in obscure encephalopathy or leukoencephalopathy; diagnosis by autoantibodies; one report of oligoclonal banding in CSF and serum[39]
Cobalamin (B$_{12}$) deficiency or dysmetabolism	Acquired B$_{12}$ deficiency or metabolic defects may cause progressive myelopathy (especially posterior and lateral columns) and peripheral neuropathy with/without overt anemia; deficits may become	Complete blood count and RBC indices; serum B$_{12}$ (low or low-normal)	M: transient T2I in cerebrum or spinal cord reported; resolve with B$_{12}$ replacement[65]	High-risk groups include patients with atypical MS, malabsorption, or GI resection or personal/family history suggestive of pernicious anemia or B$_{12}$ metabolism defect[255]; evaluate

				with serum methylmalonic acid and homocysteine (increased with B$_{12}$ insufficiency), folate[97,135,141]
	apparent after abuse or exposure to nitrous oxide			
Folate deficiency or dysmetabolism	Acquired deficiency or inborn error such as MTHFR mutation may cause progressive myelopathy, diplopia, incoordination, paresthesias misdiagnosed as MS	Complete blood count and RBC indices, serum folate	M: periventricular WM T2I described[255]	Definitive testing by serum methylmalonic acid, serum homocysteine, and specific ezyme assays (eg, MTHFR)[142]
Gluten sensitivity (celiac disease [CD] or sprue)	Autoimmune response to ingested gluten, possibly endogenous antigens, associated CD (small bowel mucosal abnormalities, malabsorption) and neurological dysfunction (relapsing-remitting or progressive ataxia is prominent; brain stem signs, peripheral neuropathy are also seen)	Antibodies to gliadin; HLA testing; small-bowel biopsy if indicated (CD symptoms)	L to M: early in disease, enhancing and T2I lesions are seen in periventricular WM and brain stem; later brain stem, cerebellar, or cerebral atrophy is observed[132]	CD-associated neurological syndrome is still being defined; CSF reportedly normal, except for antigliadin antibodies; HLA-DQ2 is found in 90% of CD patients, only 25% of normal population[150,283]

Continued

Disease	Features	Screening	MRI	Comments
Motor neuron disease	Early involvement with upper motor neuron signs alone (eg, spastic paraparesis, primary lateral sclerosis) may mimic progressive MS; rarely, MS may be associated with lower motor neuron signs such as wasting, presumably by interrupting intraspinal reflex arcs	EMG shows denervation and reinnervation affecting multiple root distributions in at least three limbs	L: MRI should be normal	Muscle wasting is occasionally seen in MS, usually in advanced cases, presumably as a result of pressure palsies or interruption of the spinal reflex arc; rarely MS and motor neuron disease have been reported to co-exist[229]

Abbreviations and Key: See Table 5.10A.

114

TABLE 5.12B — DIFFERENTIAL DIAGNOSIS OF MS: DEGENERATIVE—GENETIC

Disease	Features, Mode of Inheritance	Screening	MRI	Comments
Adrenoleukodystrophy 300100	XL: mutations of ALDP transporter protein leads to peroxisome dysfunction and excess of VLCFA; juvenile and adult (adrenomyeloneuropathy) onset forms may mimic MS by virtue of paraparesis, ataxia, mental changes, and relapsing-remitting or progressive course	Serum VLCFA (Kennedy Krieger, Athena), ACTH stimulation test for adrenal function	M: T2I are usually confluent but posterior location; extensive WM lesions in occipital region and splenium of corpus callosum pathognomonic[388]	Female carriers may present with milder disease misdiagnosed as MS; DNA testing is definitive, especially in carriers with intermediate VLCFA levels.[38]
Metachromatic leukodystrophy 250100	AR: deficiency of arylsulfatase A; in juvenile or adult-onset variants, clinical picture is of emotional and cognitive disturbance, gait abnormality, urinary incontinence; often PNS is involved	Blood (WBC) arylsulfatase A level; nerve conduction studies	M: symmetrical, diffuse areas of periventricular T2I[388]	Pseudodeficiency of enzyme in 7%-10% of normal population; distinction between true MLD and normals made by urinary sulfatide, DNA testing, metabolic study of cultured fibroblasts.[247,256]
Globoid cell leukodystrophy (Krabbe D) 245200	AR: deficiency of galactocerebroside beta-galactosidase; rare adult-onset variant associated with weakness, brain stem signs, paraparesis, visual failure, peripheral neuropathy	Blood (WBC) beta-galactocerebrosidase level; nerve conduction tests	M: confluent periventricular T2I with sparing of the U fibers; in adults, lesions may be limited to the cerebellum and brain stem[329,388]	PNS involvement distinguishes from MS; DNA testing definitive[93]

5

Continued

115

Disease	Features, Mode of Inheritance	Screening	MRI	Comments
Fabry disease 301500	XL: deficiency of lysosomal enzyme alpha-galactosidase with damage to endothelium (stroke, cardiac), skin (angiokeratomas), CNS (personality, painful crises, paresthesias, weakness), eye (corneal opacities)	Blood (WBC) alpha-galactosidase; skin lesions are characteristic (reddish-purple maculopapular lesions in the "bathing trunk" distribution)	H: in early stages, microinfarcts in cerebral WM may mimic MS; late stages show confluent lesions[388]	Adult onset with recurrent strokes may mimic MS; DNA testing may be useful, especially in female carriers or cases of pseudodeficiency; enzyme replacement effective[43,127]
Adult onset autosomal dominant leukodystrophy 169500	AD: may present in adulthood and mimic primary-progressive MS (presenting with loss of fine motor control or gait difficulty; autonomic dysfunction (decreased sweating, orthostatic hypotension) occurs early	CSF may be normal or may show increased protein and IgG; PNS is spared; optic nerves may or may not be involved	L: confluent WM lesions, sparing of subcortical U fibers[340]	Genetic defect and classification uncertain; several kindreds described were misdiagnosed as MS, although AD inheritance, prominent-early autonomic involvement, diffuse MRI changes should differentiate[70,255]
Organic acidemias	Usually AR with onset in childhood with intermittent episodes of acidosis and lethargy; however, there are reports of adolescent and adult patients with spasticity, fatigue, ataxia, optic atrophy, and elevated levels of urinary organic acids[255]	Urinary organic acid panel screen; confirmatory tests include enzyme assays and genetic testing in some cases	M: demyelination described, but no detailed reports are available[368]	Significance of association of elevated organic acids and MS uncertain; suspect if there is atypical or unexplained optic atrophy, acidosis, or positive family history

Spinocerebellar ataxias	Usually AD; progressive gait disturbance, incoordination, dysarthria, at least 17 distinct diseases described[367]	Strong family history, often with involvement of PNS; DNA testing commercially available (Athena)	L: usually shows atrophy, especially of cerebellum, brain stem, spinal cord; rarely, T2I lesions seen in brain stem[1,271]	—
Friedreich ataxia 229300	AR: usually with onset at puberty, absent stretch reflexes, progressive ataxia, posterior column type sensory loss in lower extremities; sometimes with optic atrophy, diabetes, dysarthria	Nerve conduction studies; DNA testing for GAA triplet expansion of FFDA gene, encoding frataxin (Athena)	L: usually normal or mild brain stem and cerebellar atrophy; WM T2I not reported[271]	Early in disease course deficits may mimic MS; recognize by prominent peripheral neuropathy, confirm by DNA testing
Olivopontocerebellar atrophy (SCA-1) 164400*	AD: progressive cerebellar deficits, typically with onset in midlife, ophthalmoplegia, pyramidal deficits; occasionally with optic atrophy and dementia (OPCA 1, see OMIM)	Nerve conduction test; DNA testing for SCA-1 mutation (Athena)	L: atrophy of basis pontis, medulla, spinal cord; mild or variable changes in cerebellum[197]	Often confused with MS, especially if family history is not available or is discounted[131,311]
Mitochondrial cytopathies, general	M: usually maternal transmission; but family history may be inapparent, AR, AD, or XL; disorders of cerebral, eye and muscle metabolism with episodic or fluctuating optic atrophy, paraplegia, ataxia	Lactic acidosis, elevated resting serum lactate (draw without tourniquet if possible, place on ice and transport to lab immediately); suspect with retinal pigmentation, cardiomyopathy, recurrent encephalopathy or strokelike episodes	M: often there is involvement of GM as well as WM; basal ganglia calcification; atrophy in cerebellum and other structures, nonspecific myelin lesions and a leukodystrophic pattern are also described[166,248]	Manifestations and course are extremely variable, due to extent of mitochondrial involvement in a given tissue; since eyes are often involved, opinion of experienced neuroophthalmologist often is helpful; definitive diagnosis via muscle biopsy, DNA testing of blood WBC, or muscle[99,257,388]

5

Continued

Disease	Features, Mode of Inheritance	Screening	MRI	Comments
Mitochondrial encephalopathy with lactic acidosis and strokelike episodes (MELAS) 540000	M: sudden episodes of visual loss, hemiparesis, ataxia, or headaches may mimic relapsing-remitting MS in a young adult; seizures and dementia may follow	Lactic acidosis, DNA testing for mitochondrial tRNA leucine gene (Athena)	M: multifocal cortical and subcortical strokelike lesions prominent on T2 and FLAIR sequences; diffusion-weighted images may differentiate metabolic (MELAS) from ischemic (stroke)[269]	Muscle biopsy may be necessary to demonstrate ragged red fibers and mitochondrial DNA mutation
Myoclonic epilepsy with ragged red fibers (MERRF) 545000	M: course and severity variable; myoclonic seizures predominate in classic cases; but mild cases may only show optic atrophy, fatigue, spasticity	Serum lactate; DNA testing for mitochondrial tRNA lysine gene (Athena)	M: MERRF usually reveals prominent atrophy affecting cerebral and cerebellar cortex, but periventricular WM T2 lesions and a MELAS-like MRI pattern have also been described[387]	Suspect with hearing loss, myopathy, cardiomyopathy; diagnosis from muscle histology and DNA
Neuropathy, ataxia, retinitis pigmentosa (NARP) 551500	M: ataxia, axonal sensory neuropathy, retinal degeneration, pyramidal signs, mental deterioration, proximal weakness	Nerve conduction tests; mitochondrial gene for ATPase 6 has point mutation (Athena)	L: although cerebral and cerebellar cortex atrophy are usually seen, a MELAS-like clinical and MRI presentation has been reported[387]	Visual and motor presentations have been confused with MS; suspect NARP when features of mitochondrial disease are present, especially prominent retinitis pigmentosa
Mitochondrial neurogastrointestinal encephalopathy (MNGIE) 603041*	M: ptosis, ophthalmoplegia, GI dysmobility, peripheral neuropathy, and leukoencephalopathy	Muscle biopsy (mitochondrial alterations); complex genetics (OMIM)	M: T2I of deep cerebral and cerebellar WM, diffuse and symmetrical[185]	MNGIE suggested by prominent GI involvement, including malabsorption; disease may start in childhood,

				but prominent neurological symptoms may present in adulthood
Leber hereditary optic neuropathy 535000*	M: subacute, usually bilateral, optic atrophy with little or no recovery; typically in males, often with other neurological features (myelopathy, ataxia, sensory changes)	Ophthalmological assessment; LHON is phenotypically and genotypically complex and is associated with 18 allelic variants; however, DNA testing is commercially available (Athena). (and 90% of cases are associated with mitochondrial mutations at base pairs 11778, 3460, or 14484 (OMIM)	H: T2I in cerebral WM may be identical to typical MS[100,388]	Differentiation may be difficult; LHON is favored in males with bilateral optic neuropathy, typical DNA abnormalities, few or no neurological signs, and normal CSF; however, an overlap syndrome has been described, often in women with DNA mutations and abnormal CSF[153,163,180]
Leigh syndrome (subacute necrotizing encephalomyelopathy) 256000*	M: usually a devastating childhood condition; rare adult cases have progressive or relapsing symptoms (oculomotor, cognitive, movement disorder) reflecting spongiosis and necrosis of deep brain structures (brain stem, basal ganglia)	Elevated plasma lactate pyruvate; mutations in cytochrome c oxidase gene and other genes (OMIM)	L: MRI is distinctive and shows prominent T2 signals reflecting necrosis in brain stem and basal ganglia[388]	Genetically heterogeneous; DNA testing promising but not commercially available

Continued

Disease	Features, Mode of Inheritance	Screening	MRI	Comments
Usher Syndrome 2769000*	AR: retinitis pigmentosa, deafness, psychological-cognitive defects, ataxia	CSF may show oligoclonal bands[219]; genetics complex (OMIM)	H: MRI may show patchy T2I in WM	Although prominent deafness and retinitis pigmentosa should distinguish from MS, clinical and MRI features have been associated with an MS-like presentation for Usher S[198]
Cerebral autosomal dominant arteriopathy with subcortical infarcts and leukoencephalopathy (CADASIL) 125310	AD: nonamyloid, nonatherosclerotic microangiopathy with predilection for subcortical WM, often associated with migrainelike headaches, steplike strokes, and eventual dementia	CADASIL DNA test (Athena); skin or muscle biopsy; CSF does not show increased IgG or oligoclonal bands[225]	H: T2I in periventricular and deep WM; no enhancement; predilection for temporal lobe[264]	Mutations identified in Notch 3 gene, 85% of which are assayed in commercial test (Athena); phenotype of variable severity; many families misdiagnosed as MS[97]
Cerebroretinal vasculopathy (CRV) 192315*	AD: rare brain and retinal microangiopathy presenting in 20s with leukoencephalopathy or CNS mass lesion; gait disturbance, dysarthria, cognitive decline	Strong family history, elevated ESR, abnormal fluorescein angiography	M: MRI or CT reports indicate periventricular lesions or a tumorlike mass[139,146,398]	Distinguished by retinal changes, normal CSF, AD inheritance
Hereditary endotheliopathy, retinopathy, nephropathy, stroke (HERNS) 192315*	AD: migrainelike headache, psychiatric disturbance, eventually with neurological manifestations (dysarthria, apraxia, hemiparesis, leukoencephal-	Gene defect under investigation, not linked to CADASIL mutation, but probably linked to CRV[268]	H: T2I in periventricular and deep WM, some of which enhance; confluence of lesions and clinically significant edema may occur	Only one (Chinese) kindred described to date; Jens[176] provide a useful summary of clinical and pathological distinctions among

				CADASIL, CRV, and HERNS
	opathy, dementia) and renal dysfunction (proteinuria, renal insufficiency)			
Wilson disease 277900	AR: copper deposition in tissues such as brain and liver; most common presentation ages 20-40 with dysarthria, incoordination, dystonia, tremor; over 20 mutations in the ATP7B gene identified; routine DNA testing impractical (OMIM)	Liver function tests, slit-lamp for Kayser-Fleischer rings; serum copper (elevated), ceruloplasm (low), urinary copper excretion (elevated) in combination; no finding reliable in isolation; liver biopsy sometimes required	M: often T2 hypointense lesions in basal ganglia; sometimes only T2I in frontal WM (confluent, asymmetrical)[8,388]	Subtle cases may be mistaken for cerebellar type of MS; Wilson disease "should be considered in any patient at any age presenting with unusual liver or neurological abnormalities" (OMIM)[45,138]
Adult polyglusan body disease 263570	AR: relentlessly progressive CNS-PNS disease manifest by gait disturbance, neurogenic bladder, sensory symptoms, culminating in dementia and peripheral neuropathy	Nerve conduction tests; peripheral nerve biopsy shows cytoplasmic accumulation (polyglucosan bodies)	M: extensive cerebral leukoencephalopathy and atrophy[213,351]	APBD has been misdiagnosed as MS, vascular dementia, extrapyramidal syndrome; mutations identified in glycogen branching enzyme gene[416]
Hereditary spastic paraparesis 182601*	Usually AD, rarely AR or XL; genetically and clinically heterogenous, characterized by slowly progressive spastic paraparesis (pure HSP), sometimes associated with optic atrophy, sensory changes, peripheral neuropathy (complicated HSP)	Usually MRI and CSF are normal and family history is prominent; spasticity and scissor gait may be out of proportion to other findings	L: typically normal or mild spinal cord atrophy; rarely T2I noted in cerebral WM[258,271]	Genetic loci for over 10 HSP variants have been identified but are not commercially available; most common mutation is linked to SPG4 locus in spastin gene[120,161,232]

Continued

121

Disease	Features, Mode of Inheritance	Screening	MRI	Comments
Porphyria 176000*	Usually AD (incomplete penetrance, episodic expression): disorder of heme biosynthesis presenting recurrent attacks of neuropsychiatric disturbance (bizarre mentation, pain, sensory symptoms, cranial neuropathies, seizures); mental changes and nonanatomical sensory complaints may mimic somatoform disorder[86]	Screening tests such as Watson-Schwartz are unreliable; if clinical suspicion exists, 24-hr urine obtained during attack should be sent for quantitative ALA and PBG which are elevated in all neuropsychiatric forms of porphyria[41]	M: may show reversible T2I lesions in cerebral WM during attacks,[194] but often lesions involve GM as well	Ordinarily porphyria is not confused with MS, but both conditions remain "great imitators" and are episodic; DNA mutations identified, but routine testing not currently practical[374]
Vitamin E deficiency or dysmetabolism 277460	AR: deficiency or metabolic defect (TTPA gene) involving vitamin E leads to spinocerebellar degeneration syndrome (ataxia, areflexia, weakness, ophthalmoplegia, retinal pigmentation)	Serum vitamin E level; vitamin E to cholesterol ratio is more specific[330]	H: may show T2I in periventricular and deep WM (few reports[386])	May mimic cerebellar form of MS: serum vitamin E should be measured in any unexplained ataxic syndrome[371]
Abetalipoproteinemia 200100*	AR: absence of several beta-lipoproteins causes abnormal erythrocytes, progressive ataxia, loss of stretch reflexes, ophthalmoplegia, retinitis pigmentosa[371]	Very low serum cholesterol and triglycerides; acanthocytes on blood smear (deformed, spike-like erythrocytes)	U: not reported	May mimic ataxic form of MS; serum lipids should be measured in any patient with unexplained malabsorption and neurologic symptoms[384]

Abbreviations and Key: See Table 5.10A.

Mode of inheritance: AD, autosomal dominant; AR, autosomal recessive; XL, X-linked; and M, mitochondrial (classically through maternal lineage, but pattern may appear to be AD, AR, XL, or variable, due to incomplete penetrance, heteroplasmy, and the contribution of nuclear genes). Genetic testing for many of these disorders is increasingly available on a commercial basis from sources such as the Kennedy Krieger Institute (below) or Athena Diagnostics (1-800-394-4493, www. athenadiagnostics.com).

* The disease is genetically complex, eg, a clinical condition for which several OMIM numbers exist, and only the most prominent is listed on this table. OMIM should be consulted directly for details.

When applicable, the OMIM number is indicated under the disease name. The OMIM is a catalog of human genes and genetic disorders written and edited by Dr Victor A McKusick and his colleagues at Johns Hopkins and elsewhere, and developed for the World Wide Web by the National Center for Biotechnology Information (www.ncbi.nlm.nih.gov/omim). OMIM provides a comprehensive review of clinical phenotype, gene defect, diagnostic strategy, treatment, and reference list for each disease. Given the frequent online updates by authoritative scientists, the OMIM entry often is the most up-to-date, definitive account of a disease. Excellent reviews of genetic disorders which may masquerade as MS are provided by Natowicz and Bejjani[255] and Cohen.[69] Leukodystrophies, including adult onset syndromes, are reviewed by Moser[247]; additional resources include the Kennedy Krieger Institute (1-888-554-2080, www.kennedykrieger.org) and the second opinion network of the United Leukodystrophy Foundation (815-895-3211). The MRI appearances of many of these diseases are discussed in the atlas of van der Knapp and Valk.[388]

5

TABLE 5.13—DIFFERENTIAL DIAGNOSIS OF MULTIPLE SCLEROSIS: ONCOLOGICAL

Disease	Features	Screening	MRI	Comments
CNS lymphoma	Primary or metastatic lymphoma in CNS in immunocompetent or immunosuppressed patients have been associated with focal lesions misdiagnosed as MS	CSF, including cytology; brain biopsy sometimes is necessary	M: 90% of CNS lymphomas present as enhancing lesions with mass effect; at times, early lymphoma may be identical to MS on MRI[9,44]	Steroid-responsiveness of lymphomas may lead to confusion with MS; suspect lymphoma when patient is unusually steroid dependent[90]; CSF usually has no oligoclonal bands and cytology may be positive for lymphoma
Intravascular lymphoma (malignant angioendotheliomatosis)	Rare lymphoma with intravascular location may cause CNS manifestations mimicking vasiculitis and, therefore, MS or SLE	ESR, skin lesions; usually brain biopsy required	M: usually infarcts or hemorrhages, although more subtle WM lesions suggestive of demyelination have been described[158,211]	Suspect in elderly individual with progressive course, strokelike attacks, headaches, confusion, high ESR, very high CSF protein
Paraneoplastic	Cancer may indirectly CNS dysfunction (opsoclonus-myoclonus, encephalomyelitis, cerebellar degeneration)	Serum antibodies such as anti-Ma2 (lung, testicular), anti-Yo (breast), anti-Hu (lung)[170]	M: usually normal or shows atrophy; rarely solitary[173] or subtle T2I in WM suggesting demyelination reported[24]	Diagnostic confusion may occur when cancer is undetected; paraneoplastic syndromes typically are progressive; CSF may have oligoclonal bands

| Leukoencephalopathy after chemotherapy or radiation therapy | Leukoencephalopathy after chemotherapy or radiation therapy may cause cognitive changes, headache, focal neurological signs | History of exposure, MRI changes | H: may show T2I in WM, suggesting active demyelination[119,332] | Usually history of cancer treatment is obvious and explains the leukoencephalopathy; however, florid MRI changes may surprise unwary, especially after levamisole or 5-FU treatment[185]; biopsy may be indistinguishable from MS[216] |

Abbreviations and Key: See Table 5.10A.

TABLE 5.14—DIFFERENTIAL DIAGNOSIS OF MULTIPLE SCLEROSIS: SPINAL CORD DISEASE

Disease	Features	Screening	MRI	Comments
Spondylosis	Spinal cord compression due to cervical spondylosis, disk disease, or other cause may result in a progressive myelopathy mimicking or coexisting with MS	Spinal MRI; CSF; visual evoked potentials (to establish nonspinal involvement in MS); CT myelography or conventional myelography may be indicated in difficult cases	Specificity and clinical correlation of any observed radiological findings must be evaluated critically to avoid false-positives and false-negatives	Approximately 10% of MS cases present as a myelopathy, often with subclinical demyelination at other sites; pitfall is coexistence of MS and spinal cord compressive disease; mechanical neck pain and cervical radiculopathy favor compressive disease[28,414]
Chiari malformation	Descent of the hindbrain into the spinal canal may cause headache, ataxia, ophthalmoplegia, nystagmus	Careful review of cranial and cervical spinal MRI for cerebellar tonsil herniation ≥5 mm below foramen magnum	L: in classic, uncomplicated Chiari malformation, WM is normal; confusion has occurred when minor, nonspecific WM T2I are overread	Asymptomatic Chiari malformation is frequent[235] but coexisting MS and Chiari malformation have been reported[363]; proposed relationship of Chiari malformation to fibromyalgia and chronic fatigue is unproven[405]

Spinal vascular malformations	Dural arteriovenous fistulas or intramedullary arteriovenous malformations may present as a progressive or episodic myelopathy	Spinal MRI (may be normal); myelography in prone and supine positions; spinal MRA or angiography may be required if high index of suspicion exists[34,92]	M: spinal cord T2I with swelling can mimic acute MS lesion	Differentiate from MS with cranial MRI, CSF (rarely, arteriovenous malformations are associated with oligoclonal bands)
Progressive necrotic myelopathy	Saltatory (stepwise) course, with painful myelopathy (prominent loss of reflexes, muscle atrophy) in absence of systemic disease or neoplasm	Spinal atrophy on MRI; exclude SLE, sarcoid, anticardiolipin antibody syndrome, retrovirus, herpes virus, vascular malformation, or other cause of progressive myelopathy	Cord swelling and T2I acutely; later atrophy; rarely hemorrhage[184]	Key to diagnosis is to rule out other causes, observe stepwise progression
Abbreviations and Key: See Table 5.10A.				

5

TABLE 5.15 — DIFFERENTIAL DIAGNOSIS OF MULTIPLE SCLEROSIS: TOXIC AND MISCELLANEOUS				
Disease	**Features**	**Screening**	**MRI**	**Comments**
Therapeutic agents	See Table 5.13 chemotherapy or radiation therapy complications; also cyclosporine, tacrolimus, amphotericin B, hexachlorophene, herbal extracts given parenterally and others have been implicated in toxic leukoencephalopathy[119]	History of exposure	L: diffuse WM T2I, often parallel to the lateral ventricles	Nontoxic etiologies must be excluded
Drugs of abuse	Toluene (intentional inhalation of volatile fumes, glue sniffing); alcoholism, cocaine, MDMA (ecstasy), heroin, psilocybin, nitrous oxide, and others[119]	History of exposure	M: diffuse WM T2I; after alcoholism and other abused substances, an increased number of focal T2I WM or reversible WM volume loss may be observed[27,128,289,359,377]	Exposure may be cryptic or overlooked; subtle MRI changes may be misinterpreted as early MS
Environmental toxins	Carbon monoxide poisoning after suicide attempt or accidental exposure, arsenic, mercury, carbon tetrachloride	History of exposure, urine collection for heavy metal, carboxyhemoglobin determination for acute carbon dioxide exposure	L: diffuse WM changes, variable severity[119]	Pitfalls may be cryptic or remote exposure, suggested by stable clinical or neuroimaging status

				Status of syndrome
Occupational exposure to solvents	Industrial exposure to organic solvents such as toluene, methanol, benzene, xylene, etc, "chronic painter's syndrome"	History of exposure; deficits correlated chronologically with putative dose-to-response relation; evidence of deficits on neuropsychological testing	L: WM changes usually less severe than with intentional drug abuse	debated[119]
Periventricular leukomalacia	While severe periventricular WM necrosis is easily recognized in preterm neonates, subtle PVL may only be symptomatic early in adulthood	History of premature birth or other perinatal injury	H: T2I in periventricular WM resembling typical MS; PVL lesions tend to be most apparent at the external angles of the lateral ventricles, with posteriorly squared ventricles and thinning of the peritrigonal WM[267,385]	—
Psychiatric disease, nonorganic disorders	Minor MRI abnormalities have been observed in routine screening of persons with major psychiatric disease	See psychiatric red flags, Table 5.7	M: subtle or marked T2I in WM have been observed in psychiatric diseases such as bipolar disorder[20,396] and conditions such as fibromyalgia or chronic fatigue syndrome[297]	MS eventually will manifest objective neurological signs (pale optic disk, Babinski sign, internuclear ophthalmoplegia, etc), not observed in uncomplicated, nonorganic disease; relatively minor MRI changes in these conditions are not correlated with objective neurological signs and tend to be invariant on repeated evaluation

Abbreviations and Key: see Table 5.10A.

5

Dividing the differential diagnosis into the specific subgroups above and assigning diseases within the subgroups are somewhat arbitrary; eg, some conditions have both inflammatory and genetic features and could be placed in either category. Nonetheless, if a patient has findings that implicate one subgroup as particularly likely, the differential diagnosis is reduced to a manageable number of diseases, and workup can be appropriately focused on these conditions. Performance of indicated screening tests will reveal a small number of conditions that are likely and for which intensive or invasive investigation is appropriate. A comprehensive description of each of the listed conditions is beyond the scope of this handbook; if a disease appears likely, consultation with standard references, reviews cited in the tables, or an appropriate specialist is recommended.

Summary of Multiple Sclerosis Diagnosis

The strategy presented—dividing patients into four diagnostic subgroups—is a matter of common sense and reflects the conscious or implicit practice of many experienced clinicians. Essentially, the "easy" patients such as those in group I (typical MS) or group II (evident non-MS) are quickly identified at onset, and management is begun without extensive diagnostic deliberation or laboratory determinations. Formal inclusionary criteria such as those of the McDonald Committee and cautionary criteria such as the red flags are useful adjuncts to the clinical impression of MS typicality and atypicality. An additional advantage to explicit diagnostic criteria is the incorporation of evidence-based findings, such as those indicating MRI sensitivity and specificity for MS. In retrospect, it has been the author's experience that *misdiagnosis of MS almost always has resulted from casual or incorrect application of diagnostic criteria, rather than inadequacies of the rules themselves.* After consideration of the straightforward group I and II patients, attention and resources can then be prioritized for the more difficult atypical patients, such as those in group III, in which MS is possible or likely, and group IV, in which an extensive differential diagnosis must be seriously considered.

In summary, with regard to the gold standard for diagnosis, the eventual development of clinically definite MS, there is strong evidence in support of the following statements concerning patients with initial presentations suspicious for MS:

- In group I patients meeting *strict* clinical and MRI criteria for MS and without any better explanation, MS is virtually certain (nearly 100% specificity for MS).

- In group II patients without typical symptoms and without objective or significant neurological signs, MS is very unlikely. In those group II patients in whom MRI studies are performed and are normal (including spinal MRI if appropriate), MS is virtually excluded (nearly 100% sensitivity for non-MS).

- For group III patients with findings suggestive of MS but not meeting strict clinical and MRI diagnostic criteria, in approximately 40% of cases it will not be possible to conclusively establish or exclude MS by all investigations at initial presentation; thus there is no alternative to careful follow-up and reassessment of this subset of patients.

- In group IV patients with significant neurological findings suggestive of a non-MS diagnosis, the non-MS disease will be found in the majority of cases on initial evaluation; in the minority of cases in which neither MS nor a second disease is apparent after preliminary workup, an extensive differential diagnosis may need to be considered.

In order to serve as a useful clinical reference, an attempt has been made to make the tables of differential diagnosis reasonably complete. The reader should be aware, however, that MS may be a great imitator and, conversely, may at times be imitated by almost every CNS disorder. Therefore, it is never possible to comprehensively list all conditions that may enter into the differential diagnosis of MS.

6

Disease-Modifying Treatment

Multiple sclerosis (MS) treatment is emerging from an era of therapeutic nihilism into a period in which medications are available that may alter the long-term course of the disease itself.

Multiple sclerosis therapeutics is a complex and fast-moving topic. This chapter will give an overview of our current understanding of disease-modifying treatments for MS by first reviewing the principal medications that have received regulatory approval and, second, by providing a suggested guide to the use of these medications in clinical practice based on MS clinical subtype. A key principle of therapy is individualization of management based on each patient's clinical characteristics, personal preferences, and observed responses to treatment. Also, it is anticipated that clinical trials in progress will provide new insights into current treatments or even lead to changes in recommended treatment protocols. In this regard, timely and objective reports of the latest therapeutic developments in MS may be obtained through the research bulletins of the National Multiple Sclerosis Society web site (www.nmss.org; select research). Recently, a distinguished panel of experts has presented clinical practice guidelines for disease-modifying therapies in MS.[419]

Approved Disease-Modifying Treatment

In the United States, there currently are five US Food and Drug Administration (FDA)-approved medications for which MS is a specific indication. These include:

- Three forms of recombinant human interferon
  - Interferon beta-1a (Avonex)
  - Interferon beta-1a (Rebif)
  - Interferon beta-1b (Betaseron)
- A synthetic copolymer
  - Glatiramer acetate (Copaxone)
- A chemotherapeutic agent
  - Mitoxantrone (Novantrone).

For simplicity of discussion with patients, these medications are often designated by trade name. Thus the first three medications, typically considered first-line agents for relapsing-remitting multiple sclerosis (RRMS), are conveniently called the "ABC" treatments, and with the recent FDA approval of Rebif, this acronym can be expanded to "ABCR." In Europe interferon beta-1b is available as Betaferon, equivalent to Betaseron.

■ **Interferons**

Interferons are naturally occurring proteins made by various cells of the body, often in response to infection. These molecules interfere with the replication of many viruses, hence the name of this class of cytokines. They are classified as type I (alpha, beta, tau, omega interferons) or type II (gamma interferon), depending on characteristics such as cell of origin, receptor usage, and chromosomal location of encoding genes.[293] Early trials in MS utilized native molecules and were based on the rationale that interferons might inhibit putative MS-associated viruses. More recent studies have used interferons produced by recombinant DNA technology and have primarily focused on the immune and cellular effects of these cytokines. Unexpectedly, type II interferons were found to be detrimental in MS,[275] while type I interferons have shown a consistent positive effect.

The mechanism of beneficial immunomodulation by type I interferons in MS is not completely understood, but may relate to production of cytokines that down-regulate inflammatory responses, to inhibition of cellular traffic across the blood-brain barrier, to production of favorable effects by direct action on glial cells, or to interference with viruses residing in the CNS.[293]

Avonex

Avonex is a form of recombinant interferon beta-1a that closely resembles natural human interferon beta, having an identical 166–amino-acid sequence and being produced in Chinese hamster ovary cells. Since the drug is generated in mammalian cells, carbohydrates are added to the interferon protein; ie, it is glycosylated. It is administered intramuscularly (IM) at 30 μg (6 million IU) once a week.

In the pivotal phase 3 study, 301 patients with RRMS were studied in a 24-month, double-blinded, randomized controlled study; a positive effect in favor of drug treatment versus control was seen in time to disability progression, reduction in relapse rate, and magnetic resonance imaging (MRI) measures (Table 6.1). Limited, retrospective analysis suggests that Avonex may diminish brain atrophy associated with the course of MS,[321] and long-term prospective studies are in progress to determine if this effect is robust and sustained. Other studies indicate that Avonex may ameliorate cognitive decline in MS.[121] Also, in a recent study of patients with a first attack of isolated syndromes such as optic neuritis, brain stem dysfunction, or transverse myelitis and whose MRI parameters suggested subclinical disseminated demyelinating disease,[171] Avonex was shown to delay the development of clinically definite MS.

TABLE 6.1 — SUMMARY OF PIVOTAL PHASE 3 TRIALS OF DISEASE-MODIFYING TREATMENTS*

Trial Criteria	Interferon beta-1a *Avonex* (Biogen)	Interferon beta-1b *Betaseron* (Berlex)	Glatiramer *Copaxone* (Teva)	Interferon beta-1a *Rebif* (Serono)	Mitoxantrone *Novantrone* (Immunex)
Dose†	30 µg (6 MIU) IM q wk	250 µg (8 MIU) SC qod	20 mg SC qd	44 µg (12 MIU) SC tiw	12 mg/m²/q 3 mo IV
Planned duration, subjects	2 yr, n = 301, RRMS	2 yr, n = 372, RRMS	2 yr, n = 251, RRMS	2 yr, n = 560, RRMS	2 yr, n = 188 RRMS, SPMS, PRMS
Relapse rate reduction (compared with placebo)	18% (32%*)	31%	29%	33%	67%
Effect on disability	37% delay in time to defined EDSS worsening	No change in mean EDSS at end of trial	Minor changes in EDSS and proportion of patients improving; other secondary disability end points not significant	No significant change in EDSS score; but treated patients had a stable IDSS (area under EDSS curve) vs worsening in placebo patients	EDSS improved (−0.13 points) in treated patients compared with slight worsening (+0.23 points) in placebo controls; Standard Neurological Status change +0.77 in controls, −1.07 in treated patients

136

Effect on MRI	Significant reduction in active lesions; total T2 lesion load less than placebo but not statistically significant at 2 years	75% reduction in new lesions; 1.1% decrease in T2 lesion load in treated vs 16.5% increase in placebo patients at 2 years	No MRI component in original phase 3 trial; subsequent controlled study of active patients showed a 35% reduction in active lesions	78% reduction in new lesions; T2 burden of disease 3.8% reduction in treated vs 10.9% increase in placebo group at 2 years	No patients with enhancing lesions, vs 16% of control patients with enhancing lesions
Extension studies	Benefit on relapse rate appears sustained at 2.5 additional years	At 2 years extension relapse rate is not significantly different compared with placebo	Mean extension of 5.5 months confirmed reduction in relapse rate	Clinical and MRI benefits continue with 2 years additional follow-up	2-Year additional observation suggests benefits continue after therapy stopped, no significant cardiotoxicity in MS patients

Abbreviations: EDSS, expanded disability status scale; IDSS, integrated disability status scale; IM, intramuscularly; IV, intravenous; MIU, million international units; MRI, magnetic resonance imaging; MS, multiple sclerosis; PRMS, progressive-relapsing multiple sclerosis; RRMS, relapsing-remitting multiple sclerosis; SC, subcutaneous; SPMS, secondary-progressive multiple sclerosis; tiw, three times per week.

* Assessment and explanation of the relative advantages and disadvantages of these medications are complex. Controversy exists among authorities with regard to the evaluation of each treatment's profile. In part, specific features of study design or confounding variables in a study may be relevant. For example, the reduction in relapse rate vs placebo in the phase 3 Avonex trial was only 18%, less than that observed in the trials of Betaseron, Rebif, and Copaxone; when only patients in the Avonex trial who entered the study early enough to complete 24 months or more of treatment were considered, the reduction in relapse rate was 32%. Controversy is particularly evident in the assessment of extension studies and secondary measures of drug effect,

Continued

6

with some authorities accepting the conclusions achieved and others raising methodological objections to these conclusions, such as selective dropout rates, posthoc analyses, and insufficient blinding. Reference sources and original trial reports (reviewed in References 53, 75, 157, 241, 262, 280, and 323; and other sources) should be consulted with regard to the details of the trials and discussion of specific controversies.

† Interferon doses for these agents are most clearly defined by weight (μg); IU or international unit measurements are influenced by differences among bioassays, standards for comparison, and drug-specific activities, and these variables have created ambiguities in the literature, making direct comparisons by IU difficult. Also "n" indicates the total number of subjects in the study. RRMS and similar designations indicate the type of MS patient studied. In trials in which multiple drug doses were compared, for simplicity of presentation, only results with the most effective dose, eventually approved by the FDA, are shown.

The role of Avonex and other interferons in secondary-progressive multiple sclerosis (SPMS) is controversial, with individual studies either showing or not showing a slowing of progression (IMPACT, SPECTRIMS, European SP Betaferon, NASP Betaseron, and other trials; reviewed in Coyle and Durelli[85]); at the time of writing, not all of these studies have been published, and the FDA has not approved interferon treatment for SPMS. The IMPACT study, comparing conventional Avonex treatment with a double dose (60 µg IM/week) in SPMS, did not show any increased clinical benefit at the higher dose.[85]

Like other forms of beta interferon, Avonex may be associated with fever, malaise (flulike symptoms), injection site pain, leukopenia, elevated liver function tests, and other side effects. In a minority of patients (<5%), these adverse reactions are sufficiently severe to necessitate discontinuation of treatment. However, in most patients, side effects are moderate or minimal. Because of occasional leukopenia or hepatotoxicity, it is recommended that a complete blood count and liver function panel be done every 3 to 6 months during treatment with Avonex or other interferons (Table 6.2).

Betaseron

Betaseron is a form of recombinant interferon beta-1b that differs from native human interferon beta by two amino acids and by virtue of the fact that the drug is produced in bacteria and therefore is not glycosylated. It is administered at a dose of 250 µg (8 million IU) subcutaneously (SC) every other day. Large controlled clinical trials have demonstrated the benefit of Betaseron in RRMS, particularly in terms of reduction of relapses and in MRI measures of underlying disease (Table 6.1).

Adverse reactions to Betaseron are similar to those noted with Avonex; additionally, Betaseron may cause local skin reactions by virtue of its being administered

Feature	Avonex (IM q wk)	Betaseron (SC qod)	Copaxone (SC qd)	Rebif (SC tiw)	Novantrone (IV q 3 mo)
Advantages	Weekly administration is convenient; demonstrated delay in progression of disability; possible beneficial effect on brain atrophy and cognition	Demonstrated clinical and MRI efficacy in patients with active disease; possible effect on progressive disease	Few side effects; reduction in relapses similar to interferons	Demonstrated clinical and MRI efficacy in patients with active disease; prefilled syringes, no reconstitution	Marked effect on relapse rate and disability in short-term studies; dramatic reduction in enhancing lesions
Disadvantages	Systemic side effects; IM not always tolerated; MRI effects may not be sustained; possible adverse effect on depression; weekly dosage may be sub-optimal (controversial)	Higher frequency of local reactions and neutralizing anti-bodies; reduction of relapse rate may not be sustained; exacerbation of depression in some patients	Daily injections; occasional systemic reactions; not effective in progressive patients; MRI reduction of enhancing lesions less robust than interferons	Frequent (tiw) injections; side effect profiles slightly higher than Avonex, similar to Betaseron; possible adverse effect on depression	Possible toxicities, including: immuno-suppression, delayed development of malignancies, cardio-toxicity
Laboratory monitoring*	CBC, liver functions prior to therapy, at 1 month, then q 3-6 months	CBC; liver functions prior to therapy, at 1 month, then q 3 months	Not routinely required	CBC, liver functions prior to therapy, at 1 month, then q 3-6 months	See Table 6.5

TABLE 6.2 — COMPARISON OF DISEASE-MODIFYING TREATMENTS

Ideal patient	Mild-moderate disease; convenience of weekly administration	Mild-moderate disease; maximal interferon effect	Early-mild disease; useful for patient who might be intolerant of side effects	Mild-moderate disease; maximal interferon effect; glycosylation possibly an advantage vs Betaseron?	Severe disease, moving to progressive phase; failure of first-line medications

Abbreviations: CBC, complete blood count; IM, intramuscular; IV, intravenous; MRI, magnetic resonance imaging; SC, subcutaneous; tiw, three times per week.

As noted in Table 6.1, comparison of advantages and disadvantages of each medication is complex and subject to controversy. Most practitioners will use all five of the disease-modifying treatments above, depending on patient clinical features and personal preferences. The author's overview of each medication and possible ideal patients for each treatment are given above; however, as indicated in the text, at this stage of our knowledge, treatment is largely empirical and must be individualized, with some patients apparently responding best to one medication.[241] Readers are referred to primary sources for a more detailed discussion of treatment issues and opinions of other authors. As indicated in text, early direct comparison trials of disease-modifying medications have become available, but they remain controversial in part because full reports have not yet been subject to peer review in all cases.

* The interferons (Avonex, Betaseron, Rebif) should be used with particular caution in patients with depression, seizures, thyroid abnormalities, or tendency to leukopenia. In the last two circumstances, regular thyroid function testing (eg, every 6 months) and frequent CBC testing should be employed. Interferon treatment should be discontinued if the patient has symptoms of liver disease or a >fivefold elevation of liver function tests.

SC. As indicated previously, the role of interferons in SPMS treatment is highly controversial and has not been definitively resolved from either scientific or regulatory perspectives.

Rebif

Rebif is a form of recombinant human interferon beta-1a that is virtually identical to Avonex in terms of amino acid sequence and glycosylation; the two drugs differ slightly in their manufacturing process and in preservatives added to the final preparation. Also, the recommended schedule for Rebif is 44 µg SC three times per week. In this regard, controversy exists as to optimal interferon dosage, eg, whether the higher weekly dose of interferon achieved with Rebif might be associated with improved efficacy; as noted, preliminary evidence from several studies (eg, ICOMIN, EVIDENCE) indicates that beta interferon formulation, dose, and administration may influence clinical benefit, with the results favoring more intensive schedules, such as those with Rebif and Betaseron.

In the Early Treatment of Multiple Sclerosis Study (ETOMS)[71] of patients with a first attack of demyelinating disease, treatment with Rebif was shown to delay the onset of a second clinical event similar to the result of the Controlled High-Risk Subjects Avonex Multiple Sclerosis Prevention Study (CHAMPS) of Avonex in clinically isolated demyelinating syndromes (see discussion that follows with regard to treatment recommendations).

■ Copaxone

Copaxone (copolymer 1 or glatiramer acetate) is a copolymer of four amino acids (glutamate, lysine, alanine, and tyrosine) combined approximately in proportion to the number of these constituents in the encephalogenic determinants of myelin basic protein (MBP).[123] Although originally expected to induce antimyelin immune responses, the copolymer was surprisingly found to be protective in an animal model of MS, experimental allergic encephalomyelitis (EAE). The mechanism of beneficial action in this animal model and in human disease is not completely understood; however, it is thought that Copaxone may be a decoy molecule at the level of antigen-presenting cells or possibly may favorably alter the activity of myelin-specific T cells.[123] Early trials and later large controlled studies showed that Copaxone, given at 20 mg SC daily to patients with relapsing-remitting disease, reduced attacks by about one third, an effect comparable to that observed with interferon treatment (Table 6.1).

In contrast to interferon treatment, very few side effects were noted after Copaxone administration, although on rare occasions patients experienced flushing and sensation of chest tightness, a benign reaction not associated with myocardial ischemia or anaphylaxis. Additionally, Copaxone has been found to improve MRI measures of MS activity, although the onset of this effect appears delayed and the magnitude of change less robust in comparison with interferon treatment.[72] In an early study, Copaxone was not found to be effective in a group of patients with progressive forms of MS, although this issue is being reexamined in current clinical trials, particularly in the context of sharply defined groups such as persons with primary-progressive MS (PPMS). Preliminary analysis of a large phase 3 study to assess the efficacy of Copaxone when administered orally in RRMS indicates that this preparation is unlikely to have a statistically significant benefit.[373]

■ **Novantrone**

Novantrone or mitoxantrone is a synthetic antineoplastic agent that has been used for over 2 decades in the treatment of lymphomas, breast cancer, prostatic carcinomas, and other malignancies.[156] The adverse-

143

effect profile of mitoxantrone was found to be less severe than that of many other antineoplastic agents, leading to the characterization of this drug as "a kinder, gentler chemotherapy." Several recent controlled clinical trials have investigated Novantrone, typically given IV at 12 mg/m^2 every 3 months, in worsening RRMS, SPMS, and progressive-relapsing multiple sclerosis (PRMS); results to date have been encouraging,[108,156,237] with a substantial impact on relapses, progression of disability, and new MRI lesions (Table 6.1).

Mitoxantrone has generally been well tolerated in MS patients; nevertheless, like all forms of chemotherapy, Novantrone may be associated with serious myelosuppression or infection. Additionally, in studies of cancer patients, this agent has been associated with two specific, serious toxicities:

- At cumulative doses of 140 mg/m^2, approximately 5% of treated cancer patients have experienced cardiotoxicity, with manifestations such as congestive heart failure or arrhythmias,[156] leading to the recommendation that total dose not exceed this limit (approximately 2.5 years of treatment)
- Therapy-related acute myeloid leukemias or other malignancies have been observed in 0.1% to 5% of oncological patients within 10 years of treatment.

Currently, there is insufficient follow-up to indicate the actual long-term risk of cardiotoxicity or malignancy following Novantrone treatment in MS patients, but to date, experience indicates that the risk of cardiotoxity or drug-induced malignancy is much lower than that in cancer patients; for example, Edan and associates[109] reported no clinically significant toxicity or leukemia in 293 mitoxantrone-treated MS patients with several years follow-up. Nonetheless, in view of potential toxicities, full informed consent to this or any other MS treatment is essential.

At this stage in our knowledge, most authorities would regard Novantrone as a promising and apparently very effective agent, but one whose use should be limited to patients who have exceptionally aggressive disease or who have failed first-line treatment. Because of current limitations on the duration of therapy, Novantrone may be most appropriate for management of a period of especially active disease, hopefully leading to the induction of remission and perhaps followed by maintenance therapy with a different disease-modifying medication.

■ **Other Promising Disease-Modifying Treatments**

In addition to interferons, copolymer, mitoxantrone, and other agents have shown promise with regard to modifying the course of MS. Intravenous immunoglobulin (IVIG), administered at relatively low doses (0.15 to 0.20 g/kg every month) in RRMS has been well tolerated and has shown positive effects on relapse rate and development of new MRI lesions comparable with the ABC treatments; higher doses and more intensive schedules may also be effective but have been associated with significant adverse effects.[114] Limitations of IVIG treatment relate to questions of optimal dose, high cost, limited supply, and adverse effects during high-dose treatment.

As a maintenance, long-term treatment, plasma exchange has shown equivocal or negative results when used in combination with immunosuppressive medications and remains a cumbersome therapy that has not shown convincing benefit when used alone.[399] On the other hand, plasma exchange has been shown to be dramatically effective during *acute* flares of MS that are not responsive to steroid treatment.[400]

Second-monthly IV methylprednisolone treatment for SPMS at a dose of 500 mg for 3 days (plus oral taper) has been shown to delay the onset of progression.[137] Low-dose methotrexate has been well tolerated and may slow the tempo of worsening in SPMS, especially with regard to upper-extremity function.[136] More intensive immunosuppression with azathioprine or cyclophosphamide has shown benefit in some, but not all, controlled studies in both RRMS and progressive patients; however, enthusiasm for these agents is limited by substantial side effects.[125] Byrant and colleagues[52] have systematically reviewed the evidence in support of immunomodulatory treatment of MS. The use of intensive immunosuppression should generally be reserved for patients in whom conventional therapy has failed, and these treatments should be administered at centers experienced in the use of this class of agents.

Suggested Treatment by MS Subtype

Clinical trials have increasingly focused on patients with a given MS subtype (Chapter 1, *Definition and Pathology*), and corresponding regulatory approvals have been issued for medications by specific subtype of MS. For example, patients with courses consistent with RRMS or SPMS may be experiencing very different pathophysiologies, and conceivably different treatments will be applicable to the two subtypes. On the basis of these considerations, it is practical to consider the treatment of MS by individual subtype.

■ Treatment of Monosymptomatic Demyelination

Classically, the diagnosis of MS has depended on the demonstration of clinical attacks that are disseminated in time and space; as indicated in Chapter 5, *Diagnosis and Differential Diagnosis*; however, advances such as MRI scanning have allowed the identification of patients with monosymptomatic demyelination; ie, persons who have had only a single clinical attack but who are at presumed high risk for the eventual development of a second attack indicative of clinically definite MS (CDMS). Usually, corticosteroids such as IV methylprednisolone are given acutely to speed recovery; however, with regard to eventual disease course, a pertinent issue has been whether early administration of disease-modifying treatment will be of benefit. The crucial investigations to date in this regard have been CHAMPS[171] and ETOMS.[71]

In CHAMPS, patients with a first acute clinical demyelinating event (optic neuritis, brain stem dysfunction, transverse myelitis) and evidence of prior subclinical demyelination on brain MRI (≥ 2 clinically silent lesions characteristic of MS) were treated with Avonex or placebo. Patients were monitored for the development of a second episode (that is, CDMS), and these findings were incorporated into Kaplan-Meier estimates of the probability of conversion to CDMS after 3 years' observation, which was 35% in the Avonex-treated group and 50% in the placebo group (Figure 6.1). These results clearly demonstrate that early treatment delays the development of CDMS; on the other hand, the steeply rising curves of both groups suggest that eventually all or most monosymptomatic demyelinating patients with active MRI scans will develop CDMS.

Another finding of importance is the absolute magnitude of delay in CDMS development associated with Avonex treatment. For example, the population of placebo-treated patients achieves a 35% probability of developing CDMS at 20 months after the first episode, while the group of Avonex-treated patients does not achieve this probability of CDMS development until 36 months after the first episode. In terms of counseling patients, these findings indicate that they must weigh the benefit of having a second clinical at-

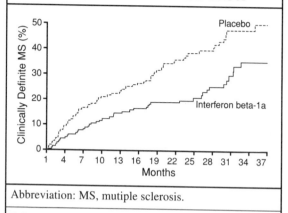

FIGURE 6.1 — CHAMPS STUDY: KAPLAN-MEIER ESTIMATES OF THE CUMULATIVE PROBABILITY OF THE DEVELOPMENT OF CLINICALLY DEFINITE MULTIPLE SCLEROSIS ACCORDING TO TREATMENT GROUP

Abbreviation: MS, mutiple sclerosis.

Reference 171.

tack delayed 16 months on average against the possible inconvenience and adverse effects of weekly interferon treatment for 3 years. Similar findings were observed in ETOMS[71] in which Rebif treatment reduced the number of patients with a first episode of neurological dysfunction suggestive of MS converting to CDMS after 2 years observation from 45% (placebo group) to 34% (treated group).

Reasonable patients and physicians may differ with regard to the treatment implications of CHAMPS and ETOMS.[107,298] It is important to keep in mind that patients seen in clinical practice will have an expected risk of developing CDMS that is either less or more than that of the patients in these investigations, carefully selected for active disease and a high risk of eventual MS. For example, prospective studies of unselected patients with the first attack of optic neuritis—a prototypic monosymptomatic demyelinating condition—have shown that as many as 48% of patients in a hospital-based practice[312] or 83% of patients in a population-based survey[284] do not develop CDMS or apparent disability after approximately 15 years of observation.[229]

At the other extreme, patients with very active MRI scans (eg, 10 to 20 total lesions, many of them enhancing), severe deficits at onset, or histories suggestive of prior, undocumented neurological events, are expected to be at exceptional risk for rapid conversion to CDMS. Another issue, not definitively resolved at this point, is whether early treatment of monosymptomatic demyelination will have a substantial, long-term benefit on neurological disability. Authorities both favoring early treatment and skeptical about early treatment agree that the benefit of treatment over decades is unknown.[71,107]

One approach to this controversy, given the imperfect state of current knowledge, is to recommend treatment with Avonex, Rebif, or possibly another modifying agent to patients who have dynamic clinical and MRI profiles and who are personally enthusiastic about active intervention. On the other hand, patients who have a lesser predicted risk of early conversion to CDMS (Chapter 4, *Neuroimaging*, and Chapter 8, *Prognosis and Management*) and who characteristically are less inclined to initiate parenteral treatment can rationally be followed by watchful waiting (Figure 6.2). In either case, the crucial consideration must be an in-depth discussion of what we currently know of risks and benefits of active treatment or watchful waiting with each patient in order to achieve truly informed consent, consistent with the patient's own preferences and with current scientific uncertainty. For patients meeting the entry criteria of CHAMPS or ETOMS, benefit should properly be pre-

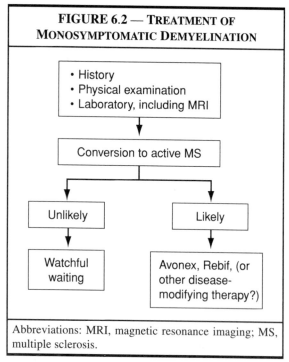

FIGURE 6.2 — TREATMENT OF MONOSYMPTOMATIC DEMYELINATION

- History
- Physical examination
- Laboratory, including MRI

↓

Conversion to active MS

Unlikely → Watchful waiting

Likely → Avonex, Rebif, (or other disease-modifying therapy?)

Abbreviations: MRI, magnetic resonance imaging; MS, multiple sclerosis.

sented as a relative delay of CDMS development, not an absolute prevention of CDMS.

■ Treatment of Relapsing-Remitting Multiple Sclerosis

Research has led to exciting breakthroughs in the treatment of RRMS, but has also generated uncertainty as to the best management of individual patients (Figure 6.3). One way to address treatment in RRMS is to consider two pertinent questions: Which RRMS patients should be recommended for therapy? Which disease-modifying treatment should be considered for a given patient?

With regard to the first issue, there is growing consensus, especially in North America, that treatment

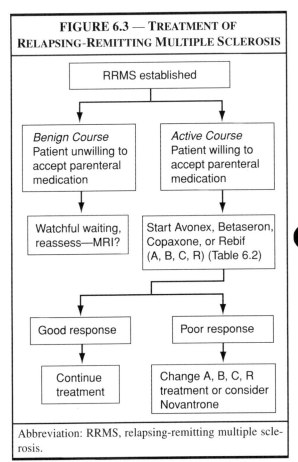

FIGURE 6.3 — TREATMENT OF RELAPSING-REMITTING MULTIPLE SCLEROSIS

RRMS established

Benign Course
Patient unwilling to accept parenteral medication

Active Course
Patient willing to accept parenteral medication

Watchful waiting, reassess—MRI?

Start Avonex, Betaseron, Copaxone, or Rebif (A, B, C, R) (Table 6.2)

Good response

Poor response

Continue treatment

Change A, B, C, R treatment or consider Novantrone

Abbreviation: RRMS, relapsing-remitting multiple sclerosis.

should be offered to virtually all RRMS patients relatively early in their disease course. This recommendation is based on firm data showing a robust effect of treatment on relapse rate and MRI parameters of inflammatory lesion development. Additionally, it is reasonable to hope that early treatment will have a significant effect on long-term tissue damage and clinical disability, and preliminary, retrospective analyses have shown favorable effects on measures such as cerebral atrophy. On the basis of these considerations, the National Multiple Sclerosis Society (NMSS) has recommended that disease-modifying treatment be given to all patients with RRMS, the first such advisory in the Society's history.

Empirical support for this advisory comes from sources such as the PRISMS-4 study,[304,342] which compared (1) RRMS patients treated with placebo for 2 years, then crossed over with Rebif treatment for an additional 2 years, with (2) patients continuously treated with Rebif for 4 years. As shown in Figure 6.4, the time to sustained disability progression was delayed by approximately 18 months in the high-dose Rebif treatment group.

Whether the 18-month delay in reaching the same disease state justifies the cost and adverse effects over 4 years of treatment depends on the clinical judgment of physicians and the informed consent of patients. As in the controversy regarding early treatment in monosymptomatic patients in CHAMPS and ETOMS, intuitively, it would seem that the "gamble" of early treatment would be proportionately attractive to RRMS patients and their physicians to the degree that their disease is active by clinical and MRI measures. In other words, for patients with active established RRMS, early treatment is a good way to gamble, to hedge one's bets; for those with inactive or minimal disease, the relative benefit of early treatment is not so clear. In this regard, the authors of a recent *New England Journal of Medicine*[262] review of MS remarked:

Opinions vary on when to initiate treatment ... Neurologists who initiate treatment when the diagnosis of relapsing-remitting multiple sclerosis is established, or shortly thereafter, believe that these drugs are maximally effective against the early inflammatory phase of the disease ... Other neurologists delay treatment until there is a his-

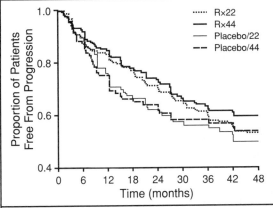

FIGURE 6.4 — PRISMS-4 STUDY: KAPLAN-MEIER CURVES FOR TIME TO CONFIRMED PROGRESSION IN DISABILITY FOR YEARS 1 THROUGH 4 (ALL PATIENTS)

Proportions of patients free from progression. The patients receiving the highest cumulative dose of therapy had the lowest rate of progression, as opposed to those receiving the lowest dose, who had the highest rate of progression. Late treatment was not associated with a catch-up to benefit of early therapy.

Patient Groups: Rx22 = 4 years treatment with Rebif, 22 mg three times/wk (tiw); Rx44 = 4 years treatment with Rebif, 44 mg tiw; Placebo/22 = 2 years placebo followed by 2 years Rebif, 22 mg tiw; Placebo/44 = 2 years placebo followed by 2 years Rebif, 44 mg tiw.

Reference 304.

tory of recurrent relapses over a more prolonged period, for a number of reasons. Patients may have a benign early course... Data on the long-term efficacy and safety of these agents are not available... The enthusiasm for these treatments, whether started immediately after the diagnosis is made or sometime later, must be tempered by

the disappointing reality that most patients con-
tinue to have relapses during treatment and ulti-
mately become increasingly disabled.

Several caveats with regard to universal treatment of RRMS are in order. First, obviously a medication cannot be administered to a patient with demonstrated allergy or severe reaction to the drug. Second, these agents are contraindicated in pregnancy, and this issue should be discussed in advance with patients of childbearing age. Avonex is listed as pregnancy risk category C; Betaseron, category C; Copaxone, category B; Rebif, category C; and Novantrone, category D.[291] (FDA pregnancy categories are based on controlled studies of the relative potential of drugs to cause birth defects, with category A being most safe, no demonstrated risk, and categories D and X least safe, positive evidence of human fetal risk.) Third, it is important to keep in mind that the pivotal phase 3 studies were performed in selected, relatively active patients at MS research centers; we do not conclusively know whether the findings of these studies are applicable to the population of patients seen in general practice, some of whom may have benign, relatively inactive, or virtually asymptomatic disease. Fourth, disease-modifying medications are approved for use in uncomplicated, clinically definite RRMS; by contrast, in patients with an atypical presentation, uncertain diagnosis, or significant medical or psychiatric comorbidity, clinical judgment is necessary to decide whether further investigation and caution regarding treatment are appropriate.

In the author's view, a reasonable approach concerning initiation of disease-modifying treatment— based on our current knowledge—is to recommend early treatment for most but not all patients with RRMS. Typical RRMS patients should be educated about the benefits, limitations, and possible adverse effects of treatment; assisted with practical aspects of drug administration; vigorously supported for insurance coverage; and encouraged to have a positive, optimistic attitude about treatment.

On the other hand, in clinical practice, MS patients will be encountered who are reluctant to consider parenteral treatment, who have complicating comorbid illnesses, or who appear likely to have a benign course (see Chapter 8). In such persons, watchful waiting is appropriate as long as the patient fully understands the risks and benefits of observation versus drug therapy, including the possibility of future attacks and disability that may or may not be preventable by early therapy. Careful monitoring, reassessment, and discussion are necessary in patients opting for watchful waiting; in such patients, often it is useful to repeat an MRI scan with contrast 4 to 12 months after initial assessment.

While treatment decisions should be primarily based on the physician's clinical judgment and the patient's preferences, certainly the MRI can provide helpful, relevant information to influence such decisions, either by demonstrating persistent stability or active subclinical disease. If subsequent clinical attacks unfortunately occur in the short term, many patients who were initially very resistant to therapy will opt for treatment and have high levels of compliance.

In the patient with RRMS, which of the available agents should be recommended? Currently, in clinical practice, monotherapy is the rule since combination therapy is not approved by the FDA, pending the results of controlled investigations. A comparison of the principal disease-modifying agents is given in Table 6.2. Novantrone currently is regarded as a second-line agent and should be reserved for patients in whom first-line treatment has failed or who have extremely aggressive disease. In part, the difficulty choosing among first-line agents (ABCR treatments) has to do with the fact that the pivotal phase 3 studies of these drugs are not completely comparable and possibly that subpopulations of MS patients may respond differently to given treatments. At the time of writing, large head-to-head, direct-comparison studies between medications (EVIDENCE, ICOMIN) have not yet been concluded or fully reported in peer-reviewed form.

Currently, there is no large, long-term, methodologically sound (blinded, randomized controls), peer-reviewed, published study that conclusively demonstrates the superiority of any of the first-line agents, although a prospective, open-label comparison of the ABC treatments over 12 months in RRMS has recently been published.[191] The authors readily acknowledge the limitations of their study design, but reasonably indicate that it was "intended to mirror the clinical practice setting in which patients are fully involved in making treatment choices"; ie, patients were given the choice of selecting no treatment or one of the ABC medications, and no statistically significant differences were noted among the four groups at enrollment. The relapse rate, defined as the mean number of attacks per patient per year in each population, was 0.97 in the untreated group, 0.85 in the Avonex group, 0.61* in the Betaseron group, and 0.62* in the Copaxone group (* = statistically significant reduction versus placebo). The percentages of patients clinically improved, unchanged, or worsened after 12 months of treatment are illustrated in Figure 6.5. The results of this investigation, as well as other research, such as the PRISMS study,[303] suggest but do not prove that the dose of interferon beta-1a achieved with weekly Avonex may be suboptimal.[261]

In the large phase 3 pivotal trials, Avonex, Betaseron, Copaxone, and Rebif each showed an approximately one third reduction in relapse rate compared with placebo (Table 6.1). Side effects of Copaxone are much less pronounced than those of the

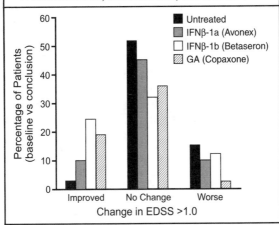

FIGURE 6.5 — CHANGE IN MULTIPLE SCLEROSIS AFTER 12 MONTHS OF THERAPY WITH AVONEX, BETASERON, OR COPAXONE

Percentage of patients who were unchanged, improved, or worse by ≥1 point on the expanded disability status scale (EDSS) after 12 months of therapy.

Reference 191

interferons, while the interferons appear to have a slightly more robust effect on inflammatory MRI lesions. These findings have led some authorities to suppose that Copaxone is more suited for patients with milder forms of MS than it is for patients with very active disease, where the interferons may offer an advantage; nevertheless, in the absence of rigorous, direct comparison studies, this recommendation is not conclusive. Copaxone also remains an attractive choice for patients who are either intolerant to or develop clinically significant antibodies to interferons.

Investigations of the three approved interferons have generally shown similar benefits and adverse effects, and it is not clear that the reported small differences among these medications will translate into meaningful, clinically significant advantages for any drug over the short or long term. In part because of the way in which it has been studied, Avonex has demonstrated abilities to delay disability and promising results with regard to retarding cerebral atrophy and cognitive decline. Also, this medication is given once a week, making it very convenient for patients with a busy work or school schedule.

Compared with Avonex, Betaseron[406] and Rebif appear to have a more striking and sustained effect on secondary biochemical measures of interferon actions, including the degree to which molecules such as neopterin are induced in healthy volunteers treated with the standard medication schedules; in this sense, Betaseron and Rebif might be regarded as "maximal interferon treatments," especially for patients with very active disease. As indicated above, there is suggestive evidence indicating that the once-per-week schedule of Avonex may be suboptimal. On the other hand, there is convincing evidence that Betaseron is more likely than Avonex or Rebif to produce significant levels of neutralizing anti-interferon antibodies, although the clinical implications of such antibodies are not clear.[293] Rebif is supplied in a prefilled syringe, a feature which is particularly helpful for patients who find reconstitution of medications difficult, and this convenient feature may soon be available for other disease-modifying medications. Both Betaseron and Rebif rarely are associated with troublesome local injection site reactions because of the schedule of frequent subcutaneous administration, a problem which is largely eliminated during once-weekly intramuscular treatment with Avonex.

Most physicians caring for patients with RRMS prescribe all four ABCR medications, depending on clinician and patient preferences (Table 6.2), as well as on the observed empirical response to treatment for at least 6 to 12 months (see the following *Individualization of Therapy* section).

■ Treatment of Secondary-Progressive Multiple Sclerosis

A suggested approach to treatment of SPMS is given in Figure 6.6. By definition, SPMS patients are those who currently have a progressive (gradually deteriorating) course and whose disease was previously relapsing-remitting (characterized only by discrete exacerbations). It should be recalled that some SPMS patients will continue to have superimposed relapses. As noted earlier in the discussion of Avonex and related medications, the benefit or lack of benefit of interferons and glatiramer for SPMS has not been conclusively determined. In the United States, the ABCR treatments are not approved for SPMS at the time of writing.

On the other hand, from a clinical perspective, it often is difficult to know precisely when the progressive phase of disease begins and predominates, ie, exactly when the conversion from RRMS to SPMS occurs. Additionally, many SPMS patients will be taking a medication originally prescribed for their disease in its RRMS phase, and, in practice, many physicians will continue this medication on an off-label basis.

Novantrone is approved for SPMS and should be considered in patients with moderate deficits who are experiencing rapid progression and who are willing to accept the potential risks of such treatment after informed discussion. Results to date with Novantrone in SPMS are very encouraging, although further experience is needed to determine the long-term benefits and risks of this form of chemotherapy. Current practice guidelines limit the total Novantone dose to 140 mg/m^2, that is approximately 2.5 years of therapy, in order to diminish the risk of cardiotoxity. Hopefully, benefit will persist beyond the treatment phase, or alter-

FIGURE 6.6 — TREATMENT OF SECONDARY-PROGRESSIVE MULTIPLE SCLEROSIS

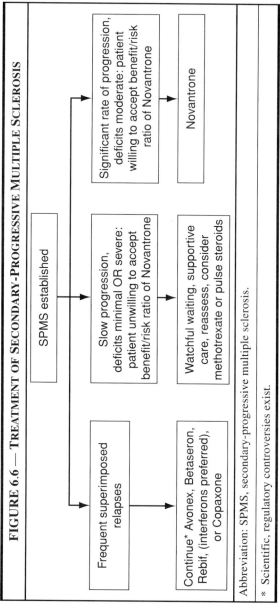

SPMS established

Frequent superimposed relapses
→ Continue* Avonex, Betaseron, Rebif, (interferons preferred), or Copaxone

Slow progression, deficits minimal OR severe: patient unwilling to accept benefit/risk ratio of Novantrone
→ Watchful waiting, supportive care, reassess, consider methotrexate or pulse steroids

Significant rate of progression, deficits moderate: patient willing to accept benefit/risk ratio of Novantrone
→ Novantrone

Abbreviation: SPMS, secondary-progressive multiple sclerosis.

* Scientific, regulatory controversies exist.

native treatment can be administered after the course of Novantrone is completed. In contrast to patients with moderate disease, patients with either severe deficits or a very slow rate of progression are unlikely to derive benefit commensurate with the risks of Novantrone treatment; in such cases, supportive care or palliative care with pulse steroids[137] or low-dose methotrexate[136] may be offered.

■ Treatment of Primary-Progressive Multiple Sclerosis

Primary-progressive multiple sclerosis (PPMS) patients represent about 10% of persons with MS. Clinical and MRI studies of PPMS indicate that this subtype may represent a distinct disease, predominantly characterized by degenerative changes such as loss of axons and oligodendrocytes, rather than the inflammatory pathology so typical of RRMS. Thus it is not clear whether basic scientific and therapeutic insights achieved in RRMS are applicable to PPMS. Currently, there is no approved treatment for PPMS, and, apart from supportive, symptomatic care, the clinician is left with the alternatives of recommending either watchful waiting, participation in trials of experimental therapy, or "off-label" use of immunosuppressive and disease-modifying agents (Figure 6.7); of the latter, perhaps Novantrone may be the most logical choice from a scientific perspective, although this currently is problematic from a regulatory perspective (please see PRMS discussion below). Clinical trials in progress may resolve these regulatory questions.

■ Treatment of Progressive-Relapsing Multiple Sclerosis

Clinically, PRMS is distinguished from PPMS by the presence of relapses superimposed on a course that otherwise has been progressive from onset. Several studies have persuasively indicated that there may be

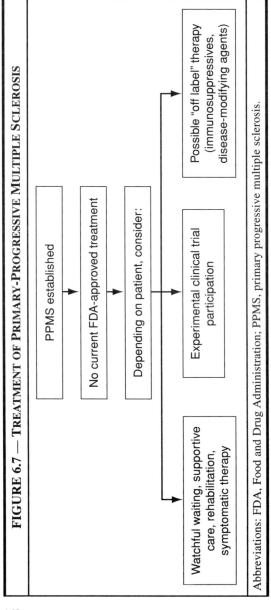

FIGURE 6.7 — TREATMENT OF PRIMARY-PROGRESSIVE MULTIPLE SCLEROSIS

PPMS established

↓

No current FDA-approved treatment

↓

Depending on patient, consider:

- Watchful waiting, supportive care, rehabilitation, symptomatic therapy
- Experimental clinical trial participation
- Possible "off label" therapy (immunosuppressives, disease-modifying agents)

Abbreviations: FDA, Food and Drug Administration; PPMS, primary progressive multiple sclerosis.

no meaningful biological distinction between PPMS and PRMS.[401] However, there is a significant regulatory reason to retain the distinction between these two disease categories, since pivotal studies of Novantrone in PRMS did show a benefit, and the medication has subsequently received FDA approval for use in this subtype of MS (Figure 6.8). Strictly, Novantrone is not approved for use in PPMS, since to date, no definitive studies of the drug in patients with this subtype of MS have been published.

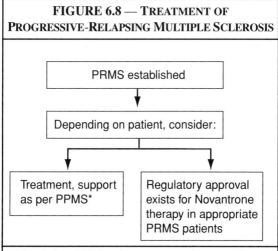

FIGURE 6.8 — TREATMENT OF PROGRESSIVE-RELAPSING MULTIPLE SCLEROSIS

Abbreviation: PPMS, primary-progressive multiple sclerosis; PRMS, progressive-relapsing multiple sclerosis.

* Current research indicates there may not be a meaningful biological distinction between PPMS and PRMS.

Individualization of Therapy

The authoritative Goodman and Gilman's text on pharmacology[259] indicates that:

... therapy as a science does not apply simply to the evaluation and testing of new, investigational drugs in animals and human beings. It applies

with equal importance to the treatment of each patient as an individual. Therapists of every type have long recognized and acknowledged that individual patients show wide variability in response to the same drug or treatment method...

From a patient's point of view, individualization also is essential. Typically, patients are not concerned with abstract statistics; usually, they ask concretely about treatment, eg, "Doctor, which medicine is best for me? If I start this treatment, what good and bad effects can I expect on my work and family life?" In responding to such questions, it is important to realistically indicate the variability of MS with or without treatment.

To illustrate patient outcomes over an intermediate time frame, results from the study of Khan and colleagues[191] and representative phase 3 studies are shown in Figures 6.5, 6.9, and 6.10. Considering each patient's progress or change from baseline status, it is apparent that there are two important sources of individual variation, even in carefully selected, relatively homogeneous experimental study populations: (1) variation in the untreated, or natural, course of MS and (2) change in disease course as a result of therapeutic intervention. Inspection of the data shows that over the time of the studies the magnitude of effect No. 1 (natural variation; distribution of outcomes within placebo population) is greater than that of No. 2 (variation due to therapy; difference between placebo and treatment populations). Specifically, by either clinical or MRI measures, a definite treatment effect was observed; nevertheless, over the period of the studies, most patients in any group were unchanged from baseline, although substantial numbers of treated patients worsened and substantial number of placebo patients spontaneously improved.

In this regard, although the results of clinical trials in MS are frequently and conveniently represented

164

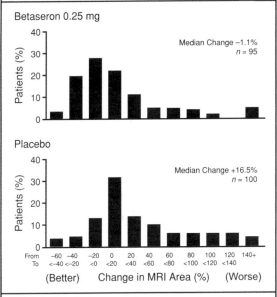

FIGURE 6.9 — BETASERON PHASE 3 STUDY: DISTRIBUTION OF CHANGE IN MRI AREA

Betaseron 0.25 mg

Median Change −1.1%
n = 95

Placebo

Median Change +16.5%
n = 100

Change in MRI Area (%) (Better) (Worse)

Abbreviation: MRI, magnetic resonance imaging.

The distribution of T2 lesion area change (baseline vs 2-year follow-up MRI) is shown.

Adapted from Reference 291.

by central measures of medication effect (eg, average, median, mean responses), the wide distribution of clinical and MRI outcomes shown in the figures indicate that excessive reliance on such measures may be misleading. This point is illustrated theoretically in Figure 6.11; note the formally trivial but clinically important truth that while the sets of data shown have identical means, they do not represent equivalent states of affairs, especially from the perspective of the dots, ie, individual patients. In Figure 6.11A, the central measure will reflect the experience of most patients,

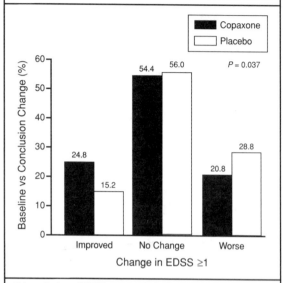

FIGURE 6.10 — COPAXONE PHASE 3 CLINICAL TRIAL: EXPANDED DISABILITY STATUS SCALE

Abbreviation: EDSS, expanded disability status scale.

The percentage of patients who improved, were unchanged, or were worse by ≥1 EDSS steps between baseline and the last (24-month) measurement in the phase 3 trial of glatiramer acetate (Copaxone). The numbers above the bars represent the percentage of patients in the respective drug or placebo group.

Reference 177.

while in Figure 6.11B, the vast majority of patients will have an outcome that is quite different from the central measure.

How, then, should patients be counseled? They should be told that in the intermediate term, their MS may improve, stabilize, or worsen, either with or without treatment. However, controlled studies indicate that treatment adds a premium, or probable increment of improvement, over and above the expected course

FIGURE 6.11 — HYPOTHETICAL POPULATIONS A AND B: CHANGE IN DISABILITY OVER TIME

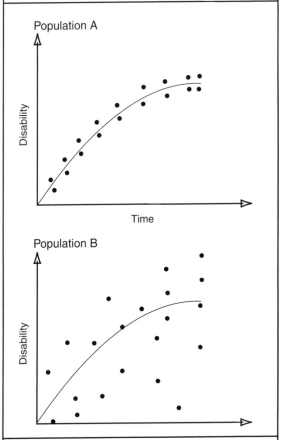

Black dots represent individual patient outcomes, ie, change in disability score as a function of time to follow-up assessment.

without treatment. MS is, unfortunately, a bit of a gamble for every patient, a roll of the dice. On the other hand, it is fortunate that treatment does influence outcome, as shown by well-controlled studies; in the gambling analogy, treatment will weigh the dice, to some extent, in the patient's favor.

Frankly discussing individual variation in disease course is important in order to dispel misunderstanding, foster realistic expectations, and thus hopefully improve compliance and satisfaction with treatment. A clear understanding of treatment effects in this variable and often unpredictable condition will better prepare patients and will encourage them to continue with therapy through the vicissitudes of their disease.

Given the heterogeneity of MS, the absence of a reliable, practical biological marker for disease activity, and our evolving knowledge of disease-modifying agents, treatment must be adjusted on an individual, empirical basis. In this regard, a series of informative patients from clinical practice are presented in Table 6.3. While none of the cases represent a scientific observation, these patients do illustrate common issues and dilemmas that will be encountered by any physician caring for patients with MS.

Patient A has had a remarkably benign course, and it is hard to imagine that disease-modifying treatment, even if available at the onset of his illness, would have improved his eventual status; on the contrary, it is likely that such treatment would only have added inconvenience and adverse effects to his long and relatively healthy life. In this regard, many individuals may have minimal or inapparent MS,[111,134,159,262] and extrapolations from autopsy series have suggested that the incidence of mild or unsuspected MS may be of the same order of magnitude as clinically active MS.[159] Such individuals, not frequently identified in the past and not prominently represented in prior natural history studies, may be increasingly coming to medical

168

attention because of increased referral to specialists and early investigation of minor symptoms with MRI scanning. It is not at all clear that conclusions derived from the study of classic MS patients selected for active disease are fully applicable to benign or virtually asymptomatic cases.

In contrast to the course of patient A, patient B illustrates that a person whose disease is relatively stable in the first few years may eventually experience fulminant exacerbation and limited recovery. Although the explosive course of patient B is exceptional, and statistically disease-modifying treatment might have been expected to only have a 30% chance of preventing her severe relapse, the possibility of a sudden, devastating attack should be borne in mind by any patient or physician opting for a strategy of watchful waiting without disease-modifying therapy. As indicated above, in the author's opinion, watchful waiting remains a rational and valid management strategy for selected patients with RRMS, but only on the assumption that their course appears to be relatively benign and that full informed consent has been achieved with regard to the relative short- and long-term risks and benefits of waiting versus treatment, based on current knowledge.

Patients C and D represent persons who apparently did better on copolymer or interferon treatment, respectively. Of course at the level of individual patients, a kind of "Heisenberg clinical uncertainty" principle operates, where it is possible to know a patient's outcome with either of two treatments, but not both simultaneously. Nevertheless, natural history studies have indicated that the average relapse rate in early RRMS is expected to be approximately one attack per patient per year. Thus it is reasonable to consider patients' treatment failures and at least raise the possibility of medication change if they experience two or three attacks, poor recovery, or persisting substantial

TABLE 6.3 — INSTRUCTIVE PATIENT EXAMPLES

	Patient Description	Treatment Course	Possible Clinical Implications
A	81-year-old man, massage therapist	51-Year course of RRMS and SPMS (MRI-confirmed), with minimal residual oculomotor and corticospinal signs, not incapacitating; good ambulation with cane, excellent, high-level mentation; no treatment	Some patients may have a benign course without therapy
B	30-year-old woman, bartender	Three minor relapses, no treatment, good recovery over 2 years noted at outside clinic; followed by fourth attack with catastrophic right hemiplegia, aphasia, obtundation. Partial recovery after IVMP, IVIG, rehabilitation, and treatment with Avonex	An initial mild course does not rule out the possibility of eventual severe attacks or persisting disability
C	42-year-old woman, anthropologist	RRMS for 12 years, EDSS 3.5, started on Avonex but experienced 2-year history of continuing attacks, marked depression, incapacitating symptoms for 3–4 days after injection, all of which ceased when Avonex was discontinued; no neutralizing antibodies to interferon; stable on Copaxone since (2 years)	Some patients appear to do better on copolymer than on interferon
D	37-year-old man, businessman	9-Year RRMS, 5 years treatment with Copaxone, but with three major exacerbations and incomplete recovery (brain stem, optic nerve, cerebellum); changed to Betaseron; no further attacks, tolerating treatment well for 3 years	Some patients appear to do better on interferon than on copolymer

170

E	36-year-old woman, graduate student	6-Year history of RRMS (clinical, MRI, CSF criteria) relentless course, frequent attacks, extremely active MRI despite treatment with Copaxone, Betaseron, IVIG, IVMP, plasma exchange, corticosteroids; clinical, MRI remission on Novantrone	Some patients fail primary therapy but respond well to cytotoxic treatment
F	52-year-old man, college professor	20-Year RRMS and SPMS; early in course treated aggressively with experimental and intensive immunosuppressive therapies at MS research center. Relentless course with dementia and institutional care required; death from pneumonia	Some patients will have a relentless course, despite most aggressive therapy available
G	50-year-old woman, secretary	25-Years RRMS with accumulating deficits, SPMS, and need for nursing home care before disease-modifying therapies were available; current status: frequent infections and marked deterioration with fevers; EDSS 9	Some patients' MS is unfortunately so advanced and their condition so medically fragile that disease-modifying treatments do not have a favorable benefit-risk ratio
H	41-year-old woman, social worker	Stormy initial 2 years of RRMS, with frequent attacks, including severe optic neuritis and sensory disturbance, making typing, driving, and work problematic; complete and continued remission for 8 years on Copaxone, fully employed and normal physical and mental activities since beginning treatment; no adverse effects from treatment	Some patients appear to have a dramatic and lasting remission with disease-modifying treatment

Abbreviations: CSF, cerebrospinal fluid; EDSS, expanded disability status scale; IVIG, intravenous immunoglobulin; IVMP, intravenous methylprednisolone; MRI, magnetic resonance imaging; MS, multiple sclerosis; RRMS, relapsing-remitting multiple sclerosis; SPMS, secondary-progressive multiple sclerosis.

6

adverse drug effects during a period of 6 to 12 months of compliance with a given medication.

Initial studies of patients treated with interferon beta indicated that the development of neutralizing antibodies to this medication may be associated with a loss of clinical response. The occurrence of such antibodies appears to be higher after Betaseron, compared with Avonex or Rebif. However, further studies have indicated that the relationship of neutralizing antibodies to interferon treatment is complex with regard to technical aspects of antibody assays, patient response to medication, and implications for changing therapy.[277] Further research is required to clarify these issues, and currently there is insufficient evidence to justify routine testing for neutralizing antibodies in asymptomatic patients or automatic cessation of treatment when such antibodies are detected.[293] On the other hand, many clinicians would consider a change of treatment, perhaps to Copaxone, in interferon beta–treated patients who develop features such as substantial worsening of their MS, clinical or biochemical evidence of toxicity after treatment (eg, fever, markedly elevated liver function tests), or very high titers of neutralizing antibodies (eg, >1:60, NabFeron assay, Athena Laboratories).

Patient E demonstrates a setting in which cytotoxic, immunosuppressive treatment was successful, while patient F unfortunately experienced a relentless course, despite the most intensive treatment available. Patient G also indicates that patients with severe, advanced disease do not typically experience a favorable benefit-risk ratio from available disease-modifying treatments, although restorative treatments under development, such as transplantation of oligodendrocytes or stem cells, may help such patients in the future. Fortunately, there are a significant number of patients like H, whose disease becomes essentially stable or quiescent after treatment. Although it is not clear whether patient H's remission is due to coincidence or to a particularly robust biological response to the treatment, certainly such outcomes are gratifying both to patients and physicians, and they are grounds for optimism and a positive attitude during discussion of proposed treatment with new patients.

Practical Aspects of Medication Administration

The manufacturers of ABCR and Novantrone disease-modifying treatments for MS supply free patient-oriented videotapes that explain drug actions, benefits, and adverse effects in lay terms. These materials are reasonably objective and directly address practical matters of patient concern, such as the details of drug reconstitution or self-administration by SC or IM means. In addition to providing didactic information, the videotapes often "break the ice" emotionally for patients in terms of comfort with chronic parenteral self-administration of drug treatment. In fact, after viewing these materials, many patients acquire a sense of participation and empowerment with regard to their treatment.

As indicated in the preceding discussion of individualization of therapy, some patients appear to respond best to Avonex, Betaseron, Copaxone, or Rebif. It is the author's practice to discuss all four medications with each patient after a diagnosis of clinically definite RRMS has been achieved; also, the role of Novantrone, typically as a second-line treatment, is mentioned. Our clinic maintains a stock of educational videotapes, supplied gratis, and, after their clinic visit, patients are asked to review materials pertaining to these treatments. At the second clinic visit or in a subsequent conversation, the relative advantages and disadvantages of each treatment are discussed, especially with regard to individual clinical course, associated medical conditions, and patient preferences.

Some patients are comfortable with risk-taking and are eager to initiate the most aggressive treatment possible. Other patients clearly are averse to risk, especially for uncertain or ambiguous benefit. Patient acceptance of treatment and long-term compliance is enhanced by attention to these variable characteristics and to individualized guidance, rather than a one-fits-all, paternalistic approach to treatment decisions. Often it is apparent that a given patient requires additional discussion or time before initiating treatment. Typically, patience and sensitivity to individual concerns are the most effective strategies, rather than an exadurated insistence that immediate treatment is an emergency. Attention to patient concerns and to compliance-assuring measures is important, since there is evidence that approximately 30% to 60% of patients will eventually discontinue initial disease-modifying treatment.[77,149]

Once a decision to begin a specific disease-modifying treatment has been reached, all that is required from the physician is to provide a prescription, and the patient only needs to call the 1-800 support number for that medication (Table 6.4). Thereafter, patient-support counselors will assist with insurance clearance, paperwork, patient education, and follow-up. Patients must receive the first treatment under medical supervision; instruction in proper injection techniques is typically given by the doctor's nurse or by a nurse working with the drug companies' patient-support office, after which most patients are able to comfortably practice self-administration. Periodic monitoring should be performed as indicated (Table 6.2) in patients receiving interferon treatment, although serious toxicity sufficient to discontinue treatment is very rare. No laboratory monitoring is required for Copaxone treatment.

Treatment with Novantrone requires special screening and close monitoring (Table 6.5). The manu-

Resource	Avonex	Betaseron	Copaxone	Rebif	Novantrone
Support*	MS ActiveSource	MS Pathways	Shared Solutions	MS LifeLines	OptiMSism
Telephone	1-800-456-2255	1-800-788-1467	1-800-887-8100	1-877-44REBIF	1-800-321-4669
Web site	www.avonex.com www.MSActiveSource.com	www.betaseron.com	www.copaxone.com	www.rebif.com	www.novantrone.com
Videotape	Yes	Yes	Yes	Yes	Yes
Autoinjector	No	Yes	Yes	Yes; prefilled syringes, no need for reconstitution	Medication is administered by clinic staff or physicians
Financial hardship program	Yes	Yes	Yes	Yes	Yes

TABLE 6.4 — PATIENT RESOURCES FOR DISEASE-MODIFYING TREATMENTS

* For questions regarding medications, prescriptions, injection training, reimbursement, medication distribution, personal therapy counseling

TABLE 6.5 — NOVANTRONE ADMINISTRATION

Prior to Therapy
- Discussion, oral consent
- Patient handout given, explained
- Insurance coverage confirmed
- Baseline transthoracic echocardiogram (LVEF >50%)

During Week Before Every Infusion (q 3 months)
- CBC with differential, platelet count, AST, GGT, total bilirubin, serum creatinine, urine pregnancy test (hCG immunoassay, before *each* infusion)
- Orders written, contact clinic nurse and pharmacy, appointment made and confirmed with patient
- Include orders for post-treatment symptom management
- Patient must be given official "Patient Information" handout prior to *each* treatment

During Therapy
- Dosage and administration:
  - The recommended dose is 12 mg/m^2 IV q 3 months, to a cumulative dose of 140 mg/m$^{2;}$ (recommendations may vary in the future, depending on studies in progress); optionally, some physicians give 1 g IV methylprednisolone at the same time
  - Stock mitoxantrone should be diluted to at least 50 mL in 0.9% sodium chloride or 5% dextrose; if needed, solution may be further diluted into dextrose 5% in water, normal saline, or dextrose 5% with normal saline
  - Mitoxantrone infusion should not be mixed with heparin; a precipitate may form
  - The diluted mitoxantrone solution should be introduced slowly into the tubing as a freely running IV infusion of 0.9% sodium chloride injection or 5% dextrose injection over a period of approximately 15-30 minutes
  - Care should be taken to avoid extravasation of mitoxantrone at the infusion site and to avoid contact of the solution with skin, mucous membranes, or eyes. In the event of such exposure, standard irrigation techniques should be used immediately.
  - Thirty minutes before mitoxantrone therapy, the patient may be given an antiemetic such as anzemet (dolasetron), 100 mg po or IV. If a patient experi-

ences nausea after the infusion, an oral antiemetic
may be given on an outpatient basis (prochlorper-
azine-compazine 10 mg po q 4 h; or lorazepam 0.5
to 1.0 mg po q 4 h)
- Adverse effects should be monitored
- Patient should give phone report next day

After Therapy
- Repeat CBC with differential, platelet count if patient
  has infection or abnormal bleeding
- Repeat transthoracic echocardiogram if patient is
  symptomatic or if total mitoxantrone dose reaches 100
  mg/m^2

Abbreviations: AST, aspartate aminotransferase; CBC, complete
blood count; GGT, gamma-glutamyl transferase; hCG, human
chorionic gonadotropin; IV, intravenous; LVEF, left ventricular
ejection fraction.

6

facturer, Immunex, supplies convenient patient instruction forms and work sheets for recording laboratory
data. It may be advisable to administer Novantrone in
collaboration with a local oncology clinic, where a specialized pharmacy and nursing staff, familiar with this
medication, is available. Similarly, although severe reactions to Novantrone are rare in patients with MS,
such reactions are always a possibility. For this reason, it may be wise to prospectively discuss Novantrone treatment with an oncological colleague willing
to serve as a consultant should marked hematopoietic
depression or life-threatening infection occur. Also,
Novantrone administration requires prescreening of
cardiac function, usually by echocardiography, to determine left ventricular ejection fraction (Table 6.5).

What are the options for patients in whom Avonex,
Betaseron, Copaxone, Rebif, or Novantrone treatment
is not successful or appropriate? First, it is important
to recall that at best, current therapies favorably modify
(this chapter) or compensate (see Chapter 7, *Symptomatic Treatment*) for the disabilities of MS; they do not
cure the disease. Stated differently, the current limitations of treatment are such that there unfortunately and

inevitably are patients who will worsen, despite our best efforts, and all that can be offered is supportive and rehabilitative care for such patients. Second, there are a variety of treatments (IVIG, plasma exchange, cyclophosphamide, azathioprine, methotrexate, total lymphoid irradiation, and others) that have shown promise in MS but that have not been validated by large clinical trials, extensive clinical experience, and official regulatory-insurance approval, which has been obtained with conventional treatments. Guidance with regard to these supplemental treatments in selected patients may be obtained through reference sources or by consultation with specialized MS centers or practitioners. Third, some patients may have an interest in volunteering for experimental treatment and may meet the entry criteria for ongoing trials of new agents. Further information concerning such trials may be obtained from nearby university hospitals or tertiary referral clinics, state chapters of the NMSS, or NMSS headquarters (web site www.nmss.org, select research (see Chapter 9, *Resources*).

Possible Future Therapeutic Developments

Prediction is hazardous, particularly about the future. This is especially so regarding the treatment of patients with an enigmatic disease such as MS. Nonetheless, several therapeutic developments appear likely in the near term. First, clinical trials in progress or on the horizon will soon result in what might be called the "fine tuning" of available disease-modifying treatments. Specifically, issues that will be addressed include optimum drug-dosing schedules, effects on progressive disease, and direct, head-to-head comparisons of medications. Possibly, long-term studies will indicate that the relatively minor differences noted among current therapies will be magnified with time; ie, over years, a given treatment may manifest dramatic increases in benefit-risk ratio, such that it clearly stands out as advantageous versus other medications. Optimistically, it may even be possible to develop reliable clinical or laboratory markers that will predict which treatment is most likely to be of benefit to an individual patient. Also, small pilot studies of combination therapy indicate that Avonex plus Copaxone, Avonex and azathioprine, Avonex and oral cyclophosphamide, and Novantrone plus Betaseron appear to be safe[12]; larger, definitive studies will be required, however, in order to conclusively establish safety and efficacy of combination treatment.

Second, in the intermediate future, sufficient follow-up will have accumulated, especially in the case of ABCR treatments, to address the safety and efficacy of these drugs over the long term; ie, over decades, the most appropriate time frame within which to assess the course of a chronic neurological disease. A subsidiary question is whether these treatments, predominantly studied in selected, relatively active MS patients, constitute a meaningful benefit applicable to patients with less-severe disease. To date, such treatments have been remarkably safe, and significant, late-appearing toxicity, while theoretically possible, appears unlikely.

Extrapolation from effects observed in clinical trials of several years' duration provides reasonable hope that treatments will substantially diminish clinical disability and markers of disease such as cerebral atrophy.[321,322] Despite this hope, currently there are insufficient data to definitively indicate whether the benefits of such treatments will be biologically robust and significant in terms of patients' lives over decades. Ideally, we hope for an impact of the magnitude that anticonvulsants have had on the natural history of epilepsy or that immunotherapy has had on the outcome of myasthenia gravis.

Against such hope and favorable preliminary indications, there also exists some evidence suggesting that those aspects of MS most easily demonstrated to be impacted by treatment, such as the relapse rate, may be dissociated from other manifestations of the disease, such as progressive disability; eg, Confavreux and colleagues, reporting on the course of 1844 MS patients followed for a mean of 11 years[78] concluded:

> We found that once a clinical threshold of irreversible disability has been reached (a score of 4 on the Kurtzke Disability Status Scale), the progression of disability is not affected by relapses, either those that occur before the onset of the progressive phase or those that supervene during this phase. The absence of a relation between relapses and irreversible disability suggests that there is a dissociation at the biologic level between recurrent acute focal inflammation and progressive degeneration of the central nervous system.... It also suggests that agents that have a short-term effect on relapses in patients with multiple sclerosis may not necessarily delay the development of disability in the long term.

Conversely, the demonstration of an apparently irreversible course once an expanded disability status scale (EDSS) of 4 has been reached has been taken by some authorities as a strong argument for early treatment of RRMS; ie, treatments should be given in the phase of the disease during which they are most likely to be effective.

In part, these important controversies may be answered by extension studies of patients originally participating in pivotal phase 3 clinical trials, although the validity of these investigations may be diminished by selection bias, lack of matched controls, and nonblinding. Perhaps the best measures in this regard ultimately will be socioeconomic: if disease-modifying

180

treatment has a dramatic, substantial impact on MS, then over the next decade or two, this benefit will be reflected in proportional improvements in outcomes such as the number of MS patients applying for disability benefits, requiring assistive devices such as wheelchairs, receiving the diagnosis of dementia, requiring institutional care, and the like. Recently, the MS International Federation established the Sylvia Lawry Center in Munich, Germany, an international collaborative center whose mission is to address these and other questions. For example, it is hoped that statistical analysis of natural history and clinical trial data may be used to create "virtual placebo groups" against which the long-term effects of disease-modifying treatment may be judged.[254]

Third, it is likely that improved immunomodulatory therapies will be found which are more specific and effective in their actions than current agents. Such treatments might be extensions or modifications of current approaches, based on improved knowledge of MS pathogenesis in terms of individual susceptibilities, environmental triggers, and disturbed immune regulation. Examples of such treatments, currently under investigation, include T-cell vaccination, peptide immunization, altered ligand treatment, hormonal therapy, and monoclonal antibody administration. Also, the possibility of correcting putative immunological abnormalities in MS by means of bone marrow transplantation is under active investigation; while early results have shown some promise,[54] currently bone marrow transplantation cannot be endorsed outside of carefully monitored experimental trials. As indicated, restorative treatments based on growth factors and replenishment of myelin-producing cells, including Schwann cells and stem cells, are also under intensive investigation in animal models. Early pilot human studies of reparative treatments have commenced, although it is anticipated that it will be many years, if ever, before such therapies can be transferred to clinical use. Finally, it is possible that entirely new, unconventional directions in MS therapy may result in a breakthrough or even a cure for this disease, eg, by eliminating an etiologic microbe or reversing a mechanism common to all autoimmune disease.

7   Symptomatic Treatment

Prioritizing Treatment on the Basis of Severity

In addition to the disease-modifying treatments described in Chapter 6, many medications and rehabilitative approaches have been shown to have a favorable impact on the symptoms of multiple sclerosis (MS). Familiarity with these modalities is important for clinical management. Symptomatic treatment also will foster a sense of optimism in patients, a reassurance that something practical and immediate may be done for their disease.

MS unfortunately tends to worsen with time, and consequently symptoms that were initially mild often will increase significantly during the disease course. In this regard, clinicians will often find it useful to categorize symptoms by different levels of severity, each with an appropriate degree of intervention (Table 7.1). Thus the first question is not how to treat the patient's symptoms, but whether the patient's symptoms currently require treatment. Although this approach is largely a matter of common sense, explicit attention to severity will avoid clinical pitfalls, and patients will not be overtreated or undertreated. A prioritized, practical approach to management will indicate when symptoms are of sufficient severity to warrant treatment, and in this case most patients will respond well to first-line treatment. Severe or unrelenting symptoms may require more extensive workup or referral, with consideration of second-line or invasive approaches.

TABLE 7.1 — CATEGORIZATION OF MULTIPLE SCLEROSIS–RELATED SYMPTOMS BY SEVERITY

Symptom Level	Definition	Example	Intervention
Minimal	Little or no interference with activities of daily living; symptoms less troubling to patient than inconvenience or adverse effects of treatment	Slight spasticity, not interfering with ambulation; increased tone may even be of benefit by contributing to stability	Reassurance; periodic reassessment and observation
Moderate	Significant interference with activities of daily living, disrupting work or social interactions, causing noticeable distress and discomfort for patient	Spasticity that slows ambulation, causes moderate extremity pain, contributes to fatigue, limits exercise or recreation	First-line treatment by primary physician (eg, stretching exercises, oral antispasticity medication)
Severe	Incapacitating, intractable symptoms, resistance to first-line treatment; marked limitation of physical or mental function	Spasticity that prevents transfers, makes personal hygiene difficult, causes severe pain or prolonged fixed postures of extremities	Second-line treatment or referral to speciality care (eg, muscle blockade, intrathecal treatment)

Common Multiple Sclerosis–Related Symptoms

■ **Acute Attack**

Especially in its early stages, MS is usually characterized by recurrent, acute periods of worsening designated by the synonyms relapses, attacks, or exacerbations. Acute attacks are due to new areas of demyelination that affect "eloquent" areas of the central nervous system. For research purposes, criteria for relapses have been defined, including:

- One or more new neurologic symptoms
- Objective change on neurological examination
- Duration of at least 24 hours
- Neurologic dysfunction that is not secondary to a transient infection or metabolic disturbance.[178]

Typical acute attacks include episodes such as monocular loss of vision (suggestive of optic neuritis) or loss of strength and sensation in the lower extremities due to demyelination in the spinal cord. Fortunately, most exacerbations are associated with significant spontaneous recovery over 2 to 6 weeks; nevertheless, attacks have substantial impact on patients and may result in permanent deficits. For these reasons, prevention and treatment of relapses are major parts of management of MS.

Relapses vary in their severity and responsiveness to treatment. Clearly, many patients experience minor exacerbations that are not of sufficient severity to meet the research criteria above or to warrant treatment with agents such as corticosteroids. Examples of minor attacks include mild sensory disturbances, slight dizziness, minimal clumsiness or heaviness of an extremity, slight visual blurring, pseudorelapses caused by treatable infections, and the like. These attacks typically have an excellent prognosis and may be treated with reassurance, close observation (eg, periodic telephone reports), judicious use of anti-inflammatory medications (eg, ibuprofen 200 mg po three times per day for 1 to 2 weeks), or antibiotics if an appropriate underlying infection is identified. The severity of an attack is judged by determining whether it substantially interferes with a patient's activities of daily living or functional status.

This issue has been most rigorously analyzed in the context of attacks of optic neuritis, where controlled studies[31-33,270] have indicated that minor attacks associated with visual acuities of 20/40 or better have an excellent prognosis that is unlikely to be improved with corticosteroid treatment. On the other hand, optic neuritis with visual loss exceeding this standard generally should be treated. A first attack of monosymptomatic demyelination also raises the question of the need for subsequent disease-modifying treatment.

The mainstays of treatment for significant exacerbations of MS are corticosteroids. Many questions remain concerning the optimal use of these agents (for review, see Kinkel[195]). In general, drugs such as methlyprednisolone have replaced earlier agents such as adrenocorticotropic hormone (ACTH). A significant controversy exists as to whether corticosteroids should be given by the oral or intravenous (IV) route. For example, in the large Optic Neuritis Study Group (ONSG) trial,[31] oral prednisone treatment was unexpectedly found to be associated with a higher subsequent relapse rate when compared with placebo or IV methylprednisolone treatments. On the basis of these findings, some authorities have recommended that corticosteroids only be given by the IV route, while others have questioned the applicability of the ONSG trial to attacks of MS and pointed to studies in which high-dose oral corticosteroid treatment appeared to be beneficial and safe. In view of this controversy and pending definitive studies, many clinicians have opted to generally treat attacks with IV methylprednisolone with or without oral steroid taper as outlined in Table 7.2.

On the basis of the ONSG trial and other investigations, a consensus has been reached that corticosteroids are of benefit in speeding recovery from acute attacks but have little or no effect on the eventual extent or level of neurological recovery. Thus corticosteroid treatment for acute attacks of MS is effective in terms of symptoms but only palliative in terms of the underlying disease; for this reason, and because of significant adverse side effects of these medications, corticosteroids should be avoided in minor attacks but encouraged for major attacks. In another context, there is some evidence that scheduled pulses of second-monthly corticosteroid intervals may benefit the course of relapsing-remitting or secondary-progressive MS[137,195]; nevertheless, this treatment may be associated with significant side effects, and the observed improvement is generally modest in comparison with that demonstrated with conventional disease-modifying treatments. With regard to continuous, long-term use of corticosteroids, Johnson[178] observes:

Current practice recommendations discourage the chronic use of glucocorticoid therapy in the management of relapsing multiple sclerosis. Occasional patients appear to become quite steroid-dependent and may raise therapeutic dilemmas, primarily because of the toxic or adverse effects of long-term steroid use.

Severe attacks that do not improve on corticosteroid treatment may respond to intravenous immunoglobulin (IVIG) or plasma exchange. In a landmark study, which was randomized and used sham-controls, Weinshenker and colleagues[400] demonstrated that 8 of 19 patients with steroid-unresponsive major attacks of demyelinating disease experienced a moderate or greater improvement after plasma exchange. In major

TABLE 7.2 — SYMPTOMATIC TREATMENT OF ACUTE ATTACKS		
Severity of Attack	**Suggested Protocol**	**Reference**
Minor	Reassurance; close observation (telephone reports or clinic visits), reassessment; anti-inflammatory medications (eg, ibuprofen 200 mg po tid)	Johnson[178]
Major		
First-line treatment (corticosteroid)	Methylprednisolone, 500-1000 mg in 100 mL normal saline, infuse in ≥60 minutes IV, daily for a total of 3-5 treatments; after IV methylprednisolone, optional course of oral prednisone, starting at 60 mg po/d and tapering to zero after 10 days; consider coverage with gastric protection (eg, ranitidine 150 mg bid), oral potassium (eg, KCL elixir 10%, 15 mL bid, or K-Dur tablets 20 mEq, one bid), and insomnia aid if necessary (eg, temazepam [Restoril], 15-mg tab, one or two at hs, or flurazepam [Dalmane] 15-mg tab, one or two at hs)	Johnson[178]; Kinkel[195]
Second-line treatment (IV immunoglobulin or plasma exchange)	IV immunoglobulin, 0.4 mg/kg each day for 5 days; contraindicated in patients with selective IgA deficiency who possess antibodies to IgA; treatment may be given as an inpatient or outpatient; or plasma exchange, seven treatments every 2 days for 14 days; typically each exchange will remove one plasma volume equivalent, and replacement fluid is with 5% albumin with or without normal saline; hematologic parameters (hematocrit, INR) should be monitored at the third treatment and thereafter, and fresh frozen plasma administered if coagulopathy is identified; typically peripheral IV access is inadequate for the complete course, and prior placement of a central access device is required; usually hospitalization is required because of the danger of bleeding from the central catheter and fatigue after treatment	Fazekas[114]; Weinshenker[400]
Third-line treatment (cytotoxic therapy)	Intravenous cyclophosphamide (see Frohman[125]); or IV mitoxantrone (see Chapter 6); or consultation or referral to MS center	Frohman[125]
Abbreviations: IV, intravenous; IgA, immunoglobulin A; INR, international normalized ratio; MS, multiple sclerosis.		

attacks or attacks unresponsive to corticosteroids, IVIG, or plasma exchange, cytotoxic therapy has been administered (Table 7.2).

■ Spasticity

Spasticity has been defined as a velocity-dependent increase in tonic stretch reflexes.[196] Clinically, spasticity is often apparent as an increase in muscle tone, particularly in the lower extremities, and commonly is associated with other upper–motor-neuron syndrome findings such as clonus, hyperreflexia, spontaneous muscle spasms, and extensor plantar responses. As indicated in Table 7.1, mild spasticity may not require active treatment, and increased extensor tone in the lower extremities may in fact be a positive benefit to patients who need moderate hypertonus in order to remain upright. Patients with moderate or severe spasticity often note an uncomfortable sense of leg stiffness or abnormal jumpiness of their legs, both of which may interfere with ambulation.

When spasticity begins to interfere with activities of daily living, instruction by a physical therapist in active stretching or passive range-of-motion exercises often is a beneficial first step. Additionally, many patients are helped by antispasticity medications such as baclofen, tizanidine, dantrium, diazepam, or other agents indicated in Table 7.3.

Treatment should start at a low dose of medication and gradually be titrated upward, depending on patient response. In some cases, combinations of these medications may be more effective than monotherapy. If a patient is refractory to first-line therapy, referral for consideration of injection with botulinum toxin or phenol, neurosurgical procedures such as dorsal rhizotomy, or implantation of an intrathecal baclofen pump should be considered. Although invasive approaches should be generally reserved for disabled (often nonambulatory) patients, frequently such treatment

7

TABLE 7.3 — ANTISPASTICITY MEDICATIONS

Generic (Trade) Drug	Availability	Starting Dose	Titration	Monitoring	Adverse Effects	Comments
Baclofen (Lioresal)	10, 20 mg tabs, scored	5 mg/d, initially; advance to tid	Increase total dose by 10 mg at 3-d intervals to maximum 80 mg/d total	LFTs at baseline and q 6 months thereafter	Fatigue, weakness, dizziness, nausea; rarely, hepatotoxicity	Avoid abrupt withdrawal
Tizanidine (Zanaflex)	2, 4 mg tabs, scored	2-4 mg/d; advance to tid	Increase total dose by 2-4 mg at 3-d intervals to maximum 36 mg/d total	LFTs and baseline, months 1, 3, and q 3 months thereafter	Hepatotoxicity, hypotension, sedation, dry mouth	Elevated LFTs in 5%
Dantrolene (Dantrium)	25, 50, 100 mg tablets	25 mg/d; advance to 2-4 times/d	Increase total dose by 25 mg/d at 4-7-d intervals to maximum 400 mg/d total	LFTs at baseline and q 3 months thereafter	Weakness, drowsiness, diarrhea, potentially irreversible hepatotoxicity	Weakness and hepatotoxicity may be significant
Diazepam (Valium)	2, 5, 10 mg tabs, scored	2 mg/d; advance to 2-4 times/d	Increase total dose by 2-4 mg/d at 3-d intervals to maximum 40 mg/d	Usually not required	Sedation, tolerance, cognitive impairment, potential dependence	Avoid abrupt withdrawal; often used in combination with medications above

Abbreviations: LFT, liver function test (eg, aspartate aminotransferase [AST] and alanine transaminase [ALT] panel).

Other medications that may be useful in the treatment of spasticity in multiple sclerosis include gabapentin (titrate to 3600 mg/d on 3-times/d schedule; experience is limited, but promising to date); clonidine (0.2-1.0 mg/d; hypotension, dizziness, bradycardia may be significant); clonazepam; and intrathecal baclofen.

References 23, 196, 411, 413.

7

results in dramatic improvement in the patient's quality of life. For example, after intrathecal baclofen treatment, patients may have complete relief of spasticity and may also report improvement in cognitive and other functions since high doses of oral medication are no longer necessary.

■ Fatigue

Fatigue, or an overwhelming sense of lassitude and energy depletion, is a frequent occurrence in multiple sclerosis. The etiophysiology of this symptom is poorly understood but may relate to the excessive production of molecules such as inflammatory cytokines. Patients often will respond to antifatigue medications (Table 7.4), but before embarking on such treatment, several preliminary steps should be undertaken. First, it is important to define each patient's symptoms carefully to be sure that fatigue is not confused with depression, lack of motor endurance, or simple deconditioning. Second, fatigue due to another underlying medical condition, such as hypothyroidism, anemia, adrenal insufficiency, neuromuscular transmission defect (eg, myasthenia gravis), infection (eg, mononucleosis), organ failure (eg, renal), or another serious illness, should be ruled out; usually an extensive workup is neither necessary nor productive unless specific findings suggest one of these conditions or the patient's fatigue is unusually severe and intractable. Third, many of the medications used to treat MS may be associated with fatigue or sedation; these medications include the interferons, all of the antispasticity medications in Table 7.3, oxybutynin, tolterodine, carbamazepine, sodium valproate, and tricyclic antidepressants.[411] In general, these medications should be used in the lowest effective dose, and in some instances, a drug holiday or rechallenge may be needed to clarify the role of a particular medication in the patient's fatigue. Finally, many MS patients find that

192

their fatigue will respond to a program of energy conservation (with instruction from an occupational therapist if necessary) and gentle exercise followed by cooling measures. Patients should be encouraged to sleep regular hours, plan their schedule carefully, recognize limits, pace activities, prioritize or save energy for important events, and partake of short rests or naps, if possible.[345]

■ Bladder Dysfunction

Symptoms of a neurogenic bladder, such as urinary urgency or hesitancy, are virtually universal in established MS; in fact, the lack of any urinary complaints is sufficiently unusual that the diagnosis of MS at least needs to be reconsidered in patients without relevant symptoms. Given the widespread occurrence of bladder dysfunction in MS, it is particularly important to determine severity and to follow a prioritized strategy.

Patients with early disease and mild symptoms, such as intermittent urgency, may only need reassurance and close follow-up. They should be encouraged to maintain an adequate fluid intake and to promptly report any worsening of symptoms or symptoms suggestive of a urinary tract infection (UTI). At times, a schedule of regularly timed voidings will alleviate symptoms and prevent inconvenient episodes of urgency.

Patients with significant urgency, sufficient to interfere with activities of daily living, may be treated with suppressant medications as indicated in Table 7.5, on the reasonable assumption that they are likely to be suffering from uncomplicated detrusor hyperactivity. With proper follow-up and medication titration ("start low, go slow"), most patients will respond satisfactorily, at least for the early part of their disease. It is important to remember, however, that different syndromes of the neurogenic bladder cannot be satis-

193

TABLE 7.4 — ANTIFATIGUE MEDICATIONS

Generic (Trade) Drug	Availability	Dose	Monitoring	Adverse Effects*	Comments
Amantadine (Symmetrel)	100 mg (generic, caps; trade, tabs)	100 mg bid-tid	Usually not required; check serum creatinine at onset	Insomnia, dizziness, headache, livedo reticularis, peripheral edema	Usually easily tolerated; sometimes 4-5-d drug holidays are helpful if efficacy seems lost; considered first-line treatment; adjust dose for creatinine clearance <50 mL/min
Pemoline (Cylert)	18.75, 37.5, 75 mg tabs, scored; 37.5 mg chewable	Initial 18.75 mg once daily in AM; increase daily dose by 18.75 mg at weekly intervals to maximum of 112 mg/d	Manufacturer recommends LFTs at baseline and every 2 weeks thereafter	Insomnia, weight loss, dizziness, nausea	Hepatotoxicity is rare but potentially severe and irreversible, LFT assays are essential; written consent required (see PDR)
Fluoxetine (Prozac)	10, 20, 40 mg caps	10-20 mg once in AM; increase by 10-20 mg/d every 2 weeks if necessary to maximum 80 mg/d; divide into AM and noon doses if >20 mg/d	Usually not required	Headache, nervousness, insomnia, anorexia, tremor	Useful in fatigue, even if patient does not have depression; other SSRI medications (eg, sertraline [Zoloft]) may be effective

| Modafinil (Provigil) | 100 (not scored), 200 (scored) mg tabs | 200 mg once in AM | Usually not required | Headache, nervousness, insomnia, nausea | Use with caution with history of psychosis, coronary artery disease, significant mitral valve prolapse, left ventricular hypertrophy; medication is expensive and insurance coverage may be problematic |

Abbreviations: LFT, liver function test (eg, aspartate aminotransferase [AST] and alanine transaminase [ALT]) panel; SSRI, selective serotonin reuptake inhibitor.

* Only most common adverse effects are listed in the table; consult product information or reference sources for complete listings

Other medications for which there is evidence of antifatigue effect in MS include central nervous system stimulants (eg, methylphenidate and dextroamphetamine, helpful in carefully selected cases), and 4-aminopyridine (experimental).

References 203, 345, 411.

TABLE 7.5 — MEDICATIONS FOR BLADDER DYSFUNCTION*

Generic (Trade) Drug	Availability	Starting Dose	Titration	Monitoring	Adverse Effects	Comments
Oxybutynin (Ditropan)	5 mg tab, scored	2.5 mg bid	Increase by 2.5 mg increments every 2 days to maximum 20 mg/d	Note* below; postvoid residuals in some patients	Drowsiness, constipation, dry mouth, urinary retention, blurred vision	Periodic drug holidays are suggested to determine need for therapy; use with caution in elderly and in cases where anticholingeric effects may be detrimental[†]
Oxybutynin (Ditropan XL)	5, 10, 15 mg extended-release tabs	5 mg once/d	Increase by 5 mg increments every 2 days to maximum 30 mg/d	As above	As above	As above
Imipramine (Tofranil)	10, 25, 50 mg scored tabs; caps also	10-25 mg hs	Increase by 25 mg hs increments each week, maximum 200 mg	As above	Dizziness, drowsiness, headache, weight gain, dry mouth, constipation	Other tricyclic antidepressants can be used for depression or insomnia and will secondarily be effective in controlling urinary urgency
Tolterodine (Detrol)	1, 2 mg tabs	1 or 2 mg bid	Increase/decrease, depending on symptoms; maximum 4 mg/d	As above	Headache, dizziness, blurred vision, constipation, rarely urinary retention	More expensive than oxybutynin; but more selective for bladder

Tolterodine (Detrol LA)	2, 4 mg caps	4 mg/d	Reduce to 2 mg/d in hepatic or renal failure, or if 4 mg not tolerated	As above	As above	As above
Desmopressin acetate‡ (DDAVP)	5 mL bottle nasal spray; 10 µg/ puff; or 0.1, 0.2 mg scored tabs	1-2 nasal puffs (10-20 µg) at hs, ½ dose/nostril; or 0.2 mg tab at hs	Gradually increase if needed to maximum 40 µg hs; or up to 0.6 mg in tabs at hs	Usually not required	Headaches, dizziness, nasal congestion, rare allergic reactions	Avoid overhydration during night hours; use with caution with hypertension, coronary artery disease and in patients prone to fluid or electrolyte imbalance

* First-line treatment for uncomplicated patients with presumed detrusor hyperactivity, assuming a favorable response to initial medication. In patients with complex symptoms, frequent urinary tract infections, or symptoms that do not improve or that worsen with above therapy, a complete urological assessment is essential.

† Because of possible anticholinergic effects, all medications in this table (except DDAVP) are contraindicated in glaucoma, myasthenia gravis, gastrointestinal obstruction, genitourinary obstruction, megacolon, or intestinal atony; they should be used with caution in those with hyperthyroidism, reflux esophagitis, heart disease, hepatic or renal disease, autonomic neuropathy, prostatic hypertrophy, ulcerative colitis, and hypertension. If patients are screened carefully and followed closely, anticholinergic effects usually are minimal and do not require cessation of treatment.

‡ Desmopressin (DDAVP) is most useful for patients with predominant or exclusively nocturnal urgency, such that nocturia interferes with sleep and consequently increases daytime fatigue. Typically, fluid retention and electrolyte disturbance are not evident, and DDAVP is well tolerated, provided patients are medically stable and do not have an excessive evening fluid intake.

References 98, 168, 212.

factorily distinguished on the basis of symptoms alone. In particular, a patient with detrusor hypoactivity or sphincter dyssynergia may present with urinary urgency, and rarely the treatments described here may precipitate urinary retention requiring emergency catheterization, an eventuality of which patients should be warned.

Patients not responding to the measures described or presenting with hesitancy, incontinence, or recurrent urinary infections should be referred for comprehensive urological assessment. Referral should also be sought for patients with episodes of retention, evidence of renal dysfunction, or marked medical or neurological disability. Typically, in such patients the evaluating urologist will obtain postvoid residual urinary volumes, imaging of the upper and lower urinary tracts, and formal urodynamic studies[168,212]; depending on results of testing, treatments may include second-line medications, a program of clean intermittent catheterization, intravesical medications, and, if required, surgical approaches such as suprapubic catheter placement.

When MS patients have symptoms suggestive of a UTI, a urinalysis should be performed. If findings indicate a probable infection (eg, positive leukocyte esterase, positive nitrite by dipstick, or more than 20 white blood cells per high-power field on microscopy) and symptoms are mild, patients should be treated with oral antibiotics (eg, trimethoprim-sulfamethoxazole, double strength, (160/800 mg [Bactrim, DS] one tablet twice per day, or ciprofloxacin [Cipro] 250 or 500 mg, one tablet twice per day); a 3-day course is recommended in uncomplicated infections in women and a 10- to 14-day course in men, diabetics, elderly, or persons with recurrent infections. Pregnant women may be treated with ampicillin or nitrofurantoin.[67,252,353] Patients with marked symptoms, high fever, difficulty retaining fluids, or severe disability should be considered for hospitalization and treatment with parenteral antibiotics.

If urinary infections are frequent or associated with resistant organisms, an opinion from a urological or infectious disease colleague should be sought. In the absence of a reversible structural urinary tract lesion, some specialists will recommend prophylactic antibiotic treatment with low doses of antibiotics such as nitrofurantoin or trimethoprim-sulfamethoxazole. On the other hand, most authorities do not recommend treatment of asymptomatic UTIs, particularly in patients with severe neurogenic bladder, irreversible structural disease, or indwelling appliances, since such treatment is unlikely to completely clear the infection and may simply be followed by a symptomatic infection with a resistant or highly pathogenic organism.

■ Pain and Sensory Disturbance

Pain is a frequent occurrence in established MS. As in patients without MS, the first step in management is always a careful history and physical examination, particularly to determine if the patient has a specific underlying cause for the pain. For example, MS patients, like the general population, not infrequently suffer from significant cervical spondylosis, chronic back pain, migraine headaches, gastroesophageal reflux, coronary artery disease, or other conditions for which specific therapy is indicated and may be curative. On the other hand, by virtue of lesions in pain-subserving pathways, MS often is associated with syndromes such as trigeminal neuralgia or dysesthesia in extremities. A variety of medications have been found effective for pain caused by MS (Table 7.6).

In general, treatment is empirical, with agents such as carbamazepine favored as initial treatment for paroxysmal pain and medications such as tricyclic antidepressants or gabapentin preferred for initial treatment of chronic, continuous pain. Principles of treat-

TABLE 7.6 — MEDICATIONS FOR PAIN

Generic (Trade) Drug	Availability	Starting Dose	Titration	Monitoring	Adverse Effects	Comments
Gabapentin (Neurontin)	100, 300, 400 mg caps; 600, 800 mg tabs	300 mg tid	Increase by 300 mg increments every 3 days to maximum of 3-6 g/d	Usually not required	Fatigue, dizziness	Usually well tolerated and effective in most pain syndromes
Nortriptyline* (Pamelor)	10, 25, 50, 75 mg caps	10-25 mg at hs	Increase by 10-25 mg at hs by weekly intervals to maximum 75-150 mg/d	Blood pressure and heart rate	Commonly, AM sedation, dry mouth, weight gain, constipation; rarely, arrhythmia, hypotension, urinary retention	Adverse effects often lessen after 1-2 weeks treatment; higher doses can be used for intractable pain if monitoring continues and titration is gradual
Carbamazepine (Tegretol)	200 mg tabs, scored; also carbatrol†	200 mg/d	Increase by 200 mg increments every 3-5 days, converting to bid or tid schedule to maximum 1200 mg/d	Baseline CBC, including platelets, renal, and LFTs; repeat at months 1, 3, and every 3 months thereafter	Rare but serious aplastic anemia and agranulocytosis; also rash, rash, drowsiness, dizziness, GI reactions, hyponatremia	Mild leukopenia usually requires only close monitoring, not cessation of drug; extended-release formulations exist, although 200-mg form is most convenient for titration

| Phenytoin (Dilantin) | 100, 300 mg caps (extended action) | 300 mg/d, usually in one dose | Dose may be adjusted at weekly intervals to achieve clinical response, guided by therapeutic level | CBC and LFTs at baseline, month 1 and thereafter; every 3-6 months if use is prolonged, check serum vitamin D levels (osteoporosis danger) | Dizziness, ataxia, nystagmus, rash, gingival hypertrophy, GI reactions | Therapeutic level (10-20 μg/mL) usually does not have to be monitored, unless adverse effect noted or titration required |

Abbreviations: CBC, complete blood count; GI, gastrointestinal; LFT, liver function test; MS, multiple sclerosis.

* Other tricyclic antidepressants (eg, amitriptyline, imipramine, or desipramine) may be effective in MS-related pain, especially dysesthesias. Often one tricyclic will be effective or tolerated when another is not; typically, anticholinergic adverse effects (least with desipramine, most with amitriptyline) are limiting. Additional medications that have been advocated for MS-related pain include baclofen, tizanidine, zonisamide, lamotrigine, valporate, capsaicin, nonsteroidal anti-inflammatory medications, tramadol, mexiletine, and other drugs.

† Carbamazepine also is available as 200- and 300-mg carbatrol, which is given on a twice daily schedule

References 175, 181, 222.

ment include reliance on monotherapy if possible, gradual titration to either relief or toxicity, and change to an alternative medication if initial drug is ineffective. In some patients, pain will be intractable, leading to consideration of evaluation by pain specialists, intermittent or long-term opiate treatment, or interventions such as trigger-point injections or intrathecal medication or simulators.

Two pain syndromes that are commonly associated with MS include trigeminal neuralgia and dysesthetic extremity pain. Trigeminal neuralgia is characterized by lancinating, instantaneous facial pain, often provoked by stimulation of trigger points on the skin or gums. Trigeminal neuralgia often will respond to carbamazepine, and after pain has been well controlled for 2 to 3 months, an attempt to reduce or withdraw medication gradually should be made.

If carbamazepine is ineffective or poorly tolerated, treatment with baclofen, phenytoin, gabapentin, lamotrigine, or topiramate often is successful. In medically refractory cases, a neurosurgical opinion should be obtained for consideration of radiofrequency rhizotomy or neurovascular decompression procedures. Although the latter operations are controversial in MS, in reported cases and in the author's experience, excellent results have been observed, especially in patients in whom magnetic resonance imaging (MRI) suggests trigeminal nerve vascular compression.[51,369] Results of gamma-knife radiosurgery for trigeminal neuralgia in MS have been disappointing to date.[49]

Dysesthetic extremity pain is manifest as an uncomfortable burning, prickly, or needling sensation; usually this pain can be well controlled with gabapentin or a tricyclic antidepressant. The management of pain associated with paroxysmal symptoms or tonic spasms is discussed below.

■ Ambulation and Movement Disorders

Unfortunately, MS is often associated with progressive ambulatory difficulties. For example, it is estimated that 50% of patients will lose the ability to walk independently after approximately 15 years from the onset,[105] although we are hopeful that disease-modifying treatment (Chapter 6, *Disease-Modifying Treatment*) will favorably modify this statistic. Also, MS is frequently accompanied by movement disorders, such as intention tremor. Colleagues who are particularly helpful in managing these symptoms include specialists in physical therapy, occupational therapy, and physiatry.

Routine referral of patients to physical therapy is neither necessary nor cost-effective, especially early in the course of the disease. However, at some point most patients notice ambulatory difficulties that limit activities of daily living, such as work or recreation. In this instance, referral to a physical therapist is very important, particularly for determining whether the patient's walking is safe and what precautions or compensatory strategies are appropriate. Depending on the assessment, a therapist may recommend exercises for balance retraining, flexibility, or strengthening. When spasticity limits ambulation, stretching exercises or the medications in Table 7.3 may be of benefit.

Eventually, most patients will require aids in ambulation such as an ankle-foot orthosis, cane, walker, wheelchair, or motorized scooter. Although typically such aids are prescribed or approved by the attending physician, the physical therapist is able to provide standardized testing of ambulation, as well as catalogues and expertise with regard to specific features and models that best suit an individual patient's needs. Periodic reassessment and retraining with physical therapy are of benefit to patients as the severity of their disease changes.

Occupational therapists provide essential help with the patient's upper-extremity function and living circumstances. Adaptive devices may make daily activities such as dressing, cooking, and communicating easier; in the unfortunate circumstance in which a patient has lost most upper-extremity functioning and is unable to use a telephone or keyboard, the occupational therapist or speech therapist may help the patient with alternative means of communication, such as a voice-activated computer. Several software programs exist for this purpose (eg, Drag-on). These programs already are a practical, user-friendly reality for patients, and the utility of this software will increase with new versions (see Chapter 9, *Resources*). Occupational therapists also have many practical solutions to barriers that may exist in the patient's home or work environment, and often an on-site assessment is of great value.

When driving competence becomes an issue, a formal evaluation by the occupational therapist, a neuropsychologist, or an examiner at the local department of transportation may provide an objective and definitive answer with regard to the patient's safety and appropriate limitations.[333,338] Finally, occupational therapists can assist patients with a structured program to conserve energy and to plan a typical day; together with antifatigue medications listed in Table 7.4, these measures often increase the patient's ability to participate in work and social life.

A particularly disabling symptom for patients is intention tremor of the upper extremities due to demyelination affecting cerebellar or brain stem structures. Different medications have been advocated for intention tremor, including clonazepam, primidone, propranolol, hydroxyzine, acetazolamide, isoniazid, buspirone, and glutethimide.[344,358,411] Although individual patient response to treatment is unpredictable and often a therapeutic trial of the first few agents listed is worth considering, in general, results are disappointing, and these medications may have significant adverse effects, particularly with regard to sedation. In this circumstance, it is important to help patients to maintain realistic goals and expectations, as well as to consider compensatory nonmedicinal strategies available through occupational therapy, such as immobilization and weighting, which often are of significant benefit.

Experience to date indicates that electrical stimulation, surgical ablation, or radiosurgery directed to specific deep brain areas, such as the thalamus, may be effective in medically intractable, selected MS patients with tremor; complications such as tremor reoccurrence, hemorrhage, or MS worsening occur in a minority of patients.[144,242,260,337,339]

■ Paroxysmal Attacks

Most symptoms of MS persist for several weeks as part of an exacerbation or are the more or less permanent sequelae of prior exacerbations or progressive disease. However, approximately 10% to 15% of patients will experience stereotypic, repeated brief attacks that often suggest brain stem involvement, as vividly described by Kelly[186]:

A very distinctive manifestation of multiple sclerosis that may very well occur as a first episode includes the paroxysmal attacks of brain stem dysfunction that last seconds or minutes only but which are repeated many times an hour for many days on end. In these attacks there will be a sudden onset of diplopia with or without vertigo, often with paresthesia of the face or tongue or both, with dysarthria and ataxia. During the attack the patient is virtually speechless and severely incapacitated, but when it is over there are usually no elicitable signs .... Almost diagnostic of multiple sclerosis is the way in which these attacks nearly always cease immediately when the patient starts to take carbamazepine ....

Other paroxysmal attacks have been described in which manifestations are predominantly dystonic, sensory, autonomic, or language-related, suggesting attacks do not always originate from brain stem pathology.[239,365] Often the frequency of attacks and the unusual symptomatology lead to the erroneous conclusion that they are psychogenic. Paroxysmal attacks usually respond dramatically to low doses of carbamazepine (eg, 200 or 400 mg/day), although occasionally higher doses of carbamazepine or other medications such as gabapentin, phenytoin, or baclofen are required. In unusual, intractable cases, bromocriptine or ibuprofen has been successful.[239] Paroxysmal attacks usually cease after a short period; thus typically, medication can be gradually and successfully withdrawn after several months of good control.

Paroxysmal attacks should be distinguished from other brief motor manifestations in MS patients, such as flexor spasms, sleep-related movement disorders, and typical epileptic seizures. Flexor spasms are simple motor contractions, usually in the lower extremities, often precipitated by movement or noxious stimuli, and associated with other components of the upper motor neuron syndrome, such as hyperreflexia and spasticity. Early in MS, spasms may be extensor rather than flexor. These movements often will respond to antispasticity measures (Table 7.3). Sleep-related disturbances such as periodic limb movements of sleep (PLMS: stereotypic, flexion, kicking, sleep arousals, daytime sleepiness) or restless-legs syndrome (RLS: disagreeable leg sensations prior to sleep onset, relief from walking or exercise) are common in the general population and may be difficult to distinguish from typical flexor spasms in MS. In some cases, referral for a formal sleep study may help with the differential diagnosis, which is important since PLMS and RLS respond to dopaminergic agents such as levodopa, bromocriptine, pergolide, pramipexole, or ropinirole. Alternatively, the use of agents such as clonazepam, gabapentin, baclofen, or, in the case of iron deficiency, iron supplementation, has been recommended.[66,349]

Typical epileptic seizures with tonic-clonic movements, loss of consciousness, and abnormal electroencephalograms have been reported in approximately 2% to 4% of patients with MS,[239] about twice the incidence of seizures in the general population. Presumably, seizures occur in MS because of plaques that abut or enter the gray matter; treatment with standard anticonvulsants such as phenytoin, carbamazepine, or valproate usually is very effective. Rarely, patients will have seizures as a manifestation of a glial tumor, the incidence of which is increased in MS[190,282] and the presence of which may be suspected by persistent deficits, severe headaches, or intractable seizures. In this setting, reappraisal and repeat MRI studies are indicated.

7

■ Sexual Disturbance

Saunders and Aisen[331] have conceptualized sexual symptoms in MS as:

- *Primary*, the direct effects of MS (eg, erectile dysfunction)
- *Secondary*, the indirect effects of MS (eg interference of spasticity with sexual activity)
- *Tertiary*, the social, psychological, and cultural factors affecting sexuality (eg, self-image or social isolation).

Each class of symptoms has its appropriate set of management or compensatory strategies. For example, male patients commonly complain of erectile dysfunction, and often this may be relieved by a trial of oral sildenafil (Viagra), 50 or 100 mg 1 hour prior to sexual activity, provided there are no contraindications such as use of nitrates, deconditioning, coronary artery disease, propensity for priapism, or medication interaction. If patients do not respond to sildenafil, referral to a urologist for consideration of alternative approaches such as vacuum erection devices, intracorporal injection therapy, or implantation of penile prostheses is warranted. Women may be helped by the use of water-soluble lubricants (eg, K-Y jelly) to overcome vaginal dryness; other measures that may be helpful are instructions on prolonged foreplay, alternatives to intercourse, and the use of appliances such as vibrators. Secondary sexual dysfunction may be addressed by optimization of therapy for spasticity, fatigue, and bladder function as indicated, and tertiary issues may be helped by treatment of depression and social issues as indicated in the sections that follow.

■ Gastrointestinal Dysfunction

Multiple sclerosis patients often complain of constipation. Factors proposed as explanations for this symptom include diminished neural input to the gut, diffuse metabolic effects (ie, similar to fatigue), weakened abdominal muscles, sedentary lifestyle, dehydration, diminished fiber intake, and medications that have anticholingeric effects. Occasionally, constipation may be severe and may be associated with intussusception, fecal impaction, or fecal incontinence. Holland[162] (Figure 7.1) has provided a rational, sequential approach to the management of constipation in MS. All patients should have a thorough history and physical, including rectal examination if appropriate, to assess gastrointestinal function and to survey for intussusception, irritable bowel syndrome, celiac sprue, diverticulosis, or other primary diseases. Essentially, the first step to controlling constipation due to MS is to assess the contribution that medications or non-MS diseases may have on bowel function. For persistent constipation due

FIGURE 7.1 — MANAGEMENT OF CONSTIPATION IN MULTIPLE SCLEROSIS

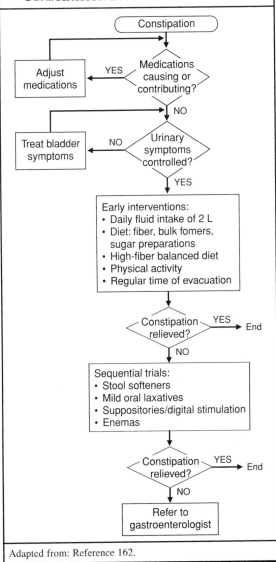

Adapted from: Reference 162.

to MS, the next step is to establish a bowel training program, the key features of which are setting a regular time of day for bowel evacuation, increasing fiber intake through food or supplements such as psyllium (Metamucil, 3 g or one single-dose packet per day with fluid), encouraging adequate hydration, increasing physical activity if possible, and using warm beverages to stimulate the gastrocolic reflex.

If constipation continues, the third step is to sequentially try agents such as stool softeners (eg, docusate [Colace] 100 mg po twice per day) or mild oral laxatives (eg, milk of magnesia 15 to 45 ml po hs or casanthranol-docusate (Peri-colace) 1 or 2 capsules at bedtime. Many patients with fecal incontinence will respond to the measures above as their constipation is relieved; essentially, regular, thorough bowel evacuation at the designated time, usually in the morning, removes the substrate for unplanned episodes of incontinence. Patients experiencing constipation, fecal incontinence, or other bowel symptoms after a conscientious effort to apply the steps above should be referred to a gastroenterological colleague.

■ Autonomic Disturbances

In addition to bladder, bowel, and sexual difficulties, MS patients sometimes experience other clinically significant symptoms referable to the autonomic nervous system, including disorders of the cardiovascular system, blood pressure, circulatory system, temperature regulation, and sweating functions. Evaluation and treatment of autonomic disorders in MS have been comprehensively reviewed by Eidelman.[110]

■ Dysphagia

The normal swallowing mechanism involves a complex interplay of neuromuscular apparatus at multiple stages, including the oral, pharyngeal, and esophageal levels. Thus it is not surprising that swallowing may be disrupted in MS patients. In general, severe dysphagia that puts the patient at risk for aspiration or malnutrition usually occurs in patients with long-standing, debilitating disease, eg, bed-bound or wheel-chair bound patients; ie, swallowing difficulties typically are proportionate to the allover level of MS disability. There may be important exceptions to this rule, however.

The key to evaluating swallowing difficulties in MS is a careful, directed history. All patients should be asked about uncomfortable swallowing, episodes of choking or coughing at mealtimes, or evident difficulty with swallowing of liquids or solids. Patients with significant symptoms should have definitive evaluation; ie, a videofluoroscopic swallowing evaluation performed by a dysphagia specialist, otolaryngologist, or gastroenterologist. Often this assessment will lead to practical aids for improved swallowing, such as changes in head position, food texture, and eating habits; in severe or intractable cases, alternative devices such as a percutaneous endoscopic gastrostomy tube may be necessary.

Obviously, it is impractical and unnecessary to perform videofluoroscopic evaluation of all patients with MS. Patients with minor or subtle symptoms may be screened by assessing lower cranial nerve functions such as the gag reflex and performing a 3-oz water-swallow test in which they are asked to drink from a cup without interruption.[96] If coughing or a post-swallow wet-hoarse voice quality is observed, patients should be referred for definitive evaluation; conversely, if patients can perform this test without difficulty, it is probable that serious neurogenic dysphagia is not present.

■ **Neuro-Ophthalmological Symptoms**

Involvement of the optic nerve, oculomotor apparatus, and other visual systems is virtually universal in MS (reviewed by Frohman et al[126]). Often consultation with an ophthalmological or neuro-ophthalmological colleague will be helpful in assessing and managing visual symptoms. Treatment of optic neuritis with corticosteroids is described earlier in the section on acute attack. Persistent diplopia may be managed by patching or special glasses with prisms. Nystagmus may be troublesome for the patient and difficult for the physician to treat; nonetheless, some success has been reported with baclofen, clonazepam, scopolamine, gabapentin, and other agents.[126]

■ Respiratory Difficulty

Occasionally, MS may be associated with acute respiratory failure. Typically, this occurs in the patients with advanced disease who are experiencing an exacerbation of MS or a significant infection with fever. Presumably, such episodes occur because of conduction block in demyelinated axons in crucial areas such as the medulla or high cervical spinal cord. With supportive care and control of underlying infection or MS flare, most patients have a favorable prognosis for return of independent breathing.[60] In the care of such individuals, it is essential to keep in mind that fever *per se* may produce failure of axonal conduction[160]; thus temperature elevations of as little as 1° to 2°C should be vigorously treated and may result in dramatic improvement in the patient's respiratory and neurological status.

Often it is difficult to determine whether patients with lesser respiratory symptoms or findings require extensive respiratory investigation and therapy. In this context, Smeltzer and colleagues[352] have developed a clinical assessment index specifically designed for respiratory screening of MS patients (Table 7.7). This index has been validated with regard to predicting expiratory muscle weakness of MS patients on formal pulmonary function tests such as forced vital capacity,

TABLE 7.7 — INDEX OF PULMONARY DYSFUNCTION IN MULTIPLE SCLEROSIS

Rating Criteria	Result	Points Assigned
Patient's Rating		
1. History of difficulty handling mucus or secretions	No = 1; Yes = 2	
2. History of cough strength	Normal = 1; Weak = 2	
Examiner's Rating		
3. Observed strength of patient's cough, after patient is asked to cough as forcefully as possible	Normal = 1; Weak = 2	
4. Number reached after patient is asked to count aloud on a single exhalation after maximum inspiratory effort	>30 = 1	
	20-29 = 2	
	10-19 = 3	
	<9 = 4	
*Total Score**		
* Total scores of 4 to 5 are considered low; 6 to 8 middle; and 9 to 11 high with regard to risk of significant respiratory dysfunction in multiple sclerosis patients.		
Reference 352.		

7

maximal voluntary ventilation, and maximal expiratory pressure. Patients with high scores on this index should be carefully monitored, especially with regard to the need for evaluation by pulmonary specialists. Early, aggressive management of respiratory tract infections, prophylactic vaccination for influenza and pneumococcus, and caution during sedation are essential.

A circumstance occasionally observed in MS and other patients is relatively subtle dyspnea or respiratory discomfort that does not appear to be associated with apparent respiratory insufficiency. Howell[165] has described such patients as suffering from behavioral breathlessness; other descriptions include disproportionate breathlessness, hyperventilation syndrome, and panic attacks associated with dyspnea.[355] Clearly, psychogenic respiratory symptoms may either occur in isolation (eg, panic disorder) or in association with underlying pulmonary disease (eg, anxiety during asthmatic attack).

Often, it can be difficult to distinguish the relative contributions of psychological and somatic factors to dyspnea; in addition to lack of obvious signs or respiratory insufficiency (Table 7.7), features that suggest a predominant role for psychological causation include dyspnea that is not related to exercise, is extremely variable in terms of symptoms or time course, is related to inspiration rather than expiration, or is associated with hot and sweaty feelings.[165] Frequently, patients with predominantly psychogenic dyspnea have a premorbid personality characterized by anxiety, resentment, bereavement, and a tendency to "catastrophize" symptoms. Such patients often are helped by cognitive-behavioral therapy and judicious use of anxiolytic medications such as benzodiazepines, antidepressants, and buspirone (described in detail by Smoller and associates[355]).

■ Cognitive and Emotional Disorders

MS is a chronic disease that has impact not only on a patient's life circumstances, but also potentially can affect almost any brain system, including those subserving cognition and emotion. Therefore, it is not surprising that many patients encounter significant mental distress at some point in their disease course. Since MS may produce these symptoms by indirect (psychosocial) and direct (brain pathology) mechanisms, it follows that both factors should be considered in planning treatment strategies.

Research has indicated that a substantial proportion of patients with MS may have cognitive dysfunction, particularly with regard to memory, abstract reasoning, attention, speed of information processing, verbal fluency, and visuospacial skills.[208,308] Often, but not always, the severity of cognitive dysfunction correlates with the general level of MS-related disability and MRI measures such as cerebral atrophy and involvement of specific brain structures, including the corpus callosum.

Determining the degree of cognitive impairment may have important implications for patient management and disability certification. For example, a patient with marked memory impairment may not be able to assimilate physician instructions, patient educational information, or efforts at vocational retraining. Also, isolated or predominant cognitive dysfunction may be a legitimate justification for granting disability benefits. Unfortunately, standard bedside testing instruments, such as the Mini Mental Status Exam, may miss approximately 50% of patients with significant deficits.[208] Definitive assessment usually requires a battery of neuropsychological tests, but in clinical practice, it is impractical to test all patients. Above and beyond the time and expense of neuropsychological assessment, many patients are fearful of testing and may be psychologically threatened by the documentation of minor abnormalities, which may have little practical impact and no effective treatment.

How, then, should patients be screened for cognitive dysfunction, and what can be done about this problem? Most important, all patients with MS should be explicitly asked about cognition. For example, a nonthreatening initial question might be, "Have you noticed any difficulty with your memory or concentration?" Follow-up questioning then can involve reports from family members, comparisons with peers of equal age and social-educational circumstances, elicitation of specific examples of cognitive dysfunction, as well as clarification of the impact of symptoms on personal and vocational life. If this inquiry reveals significant dysfunction, particularly from the perspective of the patient or family members, the subject of neuropsychological testing should be raised. Often it is helpful to frame the assessment in practical terms such as, "The psychologist can help us understand whether the memory lapses you've noticed are minor and not to be worried about or whether we need to look more deeply into this problem" or "The neuropsychological report will give us norms and objective numbers that will be important in your upcoming disability application."

Unfortunately, the management of cognitive dysfunction in MS is often less than satisfactory. Certainly, when major deficits are evident on clinical and formal assessments, disability benefits and protective measures are appropriate and should be aggressively sought on the patient's behalf. Pharmacologic treatments such as those used in Alzheimer's disease have been studied in MS, but to date these agents have not been found to be effective.[317]

Psychological efforts at cognitive rehabilitation have been either restorative (eg, memory training) or compensatory (eg, substitution of preserved abilities in specified tasks). In general, results with the former strategy have been disappointing, but the latter strategy has been reasonably effective in many patients (Table 7.8). Guidelines to compensatory approaches can be had from colleagues in mental health specialities, as well as standard references.[208,344] The treatment of factors that exacerbate cognitive dysfunction may lead to substantial improvement in mental functioning. Prominent among these factors is emotional distress.

Emotional symptoms, like cognitive changes, are frequent in MS but vary significantly in severity. For example, sadness and negative emotions are virtually universal at some point during the course of MS, and these symptoms span a continuum ranging from mild discouragement, which may be dispelled by brief reassurance from the primary caregiver, to life-threatening depression, which may require hospitalization. Several excellent resources exist to guide primary care physicians in the evaluation and treatment of depression.[327,404] All patients should be asked about mood with questions such as "How have your spirits been recently?" or "Have you noticed any problem with depression or other emotions?" Follow-up questions should address vegitative symptoms (sleep, appetitie, pleasurable goals) and possible suicidal ideation.[300]

The response to these questions should indicate the presence and severity of depression. If the depression is mild, symptoms may be managed by support and frequent reassessment by the primary caregiver and family. For some patients whose symptoms appear to center around frustration with their disease, grief for lost functions, poor coping skills, or the like, often brief counseling by a psychologist, particularly one with an interest in chronic disease or rehabilitation, may be of substantial benefit. Moderate depression, especially with vegetative symptoms, often indicates the need for antidepressant medication. Many MS patients will respond dramatically to support, encouragement, and antidepressant medication. Primary practi-

TABLE 7.8 — STRATEGIES FOR MANAGING COGNITIVE PROBLEMS

- Make lists: shopping lists, list of things to do, and so forth
- Use a calendar for appointments and reminders of special days
- Establish a memory notebook to log daily events, reminders and/or messages from family and friends*
- Use a tape recorder to help remember information or make up lists
- Organize your environment so that things remain in familiar places
- Carry on conversations in quiet places to minimize environmental distractions
- Ask people to keep directions simple
- Repeat information and write down important points
- Establish good eye contact during any discussion
- Both electronic (eg, computer) and nonelectronic organizers may be very helpful in organizing your life

* Often, consolidating all items that must be responded to in a patient's day into a memory notebook or single list simplifies cognitive effort: there is just *one* thing to remember and respond to. If unfortunately the patient frequently forgets to consult the notebook or prepared lists, often the following strategy is effective. First, the patient is provided with an inexpensive digital watch, and the watch is then set to chime at every hour during the day. Second, the patient is encouraged to develop the habit of automatically reviewing the notebook whenever he or she hears the auditory signal generated by the watch. In this way, even when alone, the patient will continuously monitor the major events, instructions, and tasks of the day by means of the auxiliary memory provided by the watch-notebook combination.

Adapted from Reference 344.

tioners are advised to develop familiarity and expertise with a small number of agents with whose use they are comfortable.

Often, a serotonin selective reuptake inhibitor (SSRI) (eg, fluoxetine [Prozac], 20 mg po q AM; paroxetine [Paxil], 20 mg q AM, or sertraline [Zoloft], 50 mg q AM, increased if needed) is considered the first drug of choice. If initial doses of the SSRI are not effective after 2 to 3 weeks, higher doses may be required; conversely, if side effects such as headache, dizziness, constipation, nausea, anorexia, or sexual dysfunction are significant, dose reduction or change to a different SSRI may be effective. Agents such as bupropion (Wellbutrin, starting at 100 mg twice a day and increasing as needed) may be effective for patients experiencing sexual dysfunction on SSRI medication; trazodone (Desyrel, 50 or 100 mg hs) may be helpful for patients with marked insomnia or concomitant anxiety.

Although tricyclic antidepressants (TCAs) such as nortriptyline (Pamelor 25 mg hs, increasing to 50 to 100 mg hs) are used less frequently than newer antidepressants in general practice because of adverse symptoms, in many MS patients, side effect such as anticholinergic actions may be desirable, eg, in controlling hyperactive bladder or excessive oral secretions. TCA medications often also dramatically improve dysesthesia and other painful symptoms.

Referral of a patient to a psychiatric colleague should be made when depression is severe, symptoms do not respond to first-line therapy, risk of suicide is evident, or the practitioner is uncomfortable with the patient's management. In severe, recalcitrant cases, electroshock therapy has been effective and safe in MS, provided no active lesions are shown on MRI scanning.[230] In addition to depression, MS patients also may experience mood swings, emotional crescendos, euphoria, antisocial behavior, sexual inappropriateness, psychotic states, and affective release (reviewed in LaRocca[208]). The latter, sometimes referred to as pseudobulbar affect, consists of brief outbursts of affective display (crying, laughing) that are not proportionate to the patient's underlying feelings; for example, a patient may experience uncontrollable crying on hearing some trivial report (eg, "Tomorrow will be cloudy"), despite little or no subjective emotional concern for this news. Affective release may be a source of severe embarrassment and social incapacitation for patients; interestingly, this symptom often responds dramatically to extremely low doses of TCAs (eg, 10 to 25 mg of amitriptyline orally every day).

Management of Complicated or Intractable Symptoms

When there is marked disability, consultation with an appropriate colleague, such as a physiatrist, neurologist with rehabilitative expertise, other specialist, or a comprehensive MS multidisciplinary clinic may be useful; at times referral for inpatient or institutional care may be required to adequately control symptoms. Some patients, especially in the middle or latter stages of the disease, may have multiple, complex combinations of rehabilitative problems that are difficult to effectively address in a typical busy clinic setting. In this circumstance, consideration should be given to referral to a comprehensive MS clinic that offers multidisciplinary patient assessment and care. An alternative, particularly in cases with severe symptoms, is to discuss brief inpatient management with a colleague in physiatry. Often a stay of only 5 to 7 days provides patients with in-depth, specialized attention to each major symptom, such that lasting improved status is manifest at subsequent routine clinic visits, as well as in the spheres of work and family life. Recent publications indicate the objective value of brief, intensive rehabilitative interventions in MS.[124] Hopefully, disease-modifying treatments may reduce attacks, disability, and the need for symptomatic treatment in MS.

8 Prognosis and Management

Multiple sclerosis (MS) is a lifelong neurological disease that is potentially disabling and for which currently there is no prevention or cure. Nevertheless, much can be done to help patients cope with MS and modify the course of their disease; in this sense, the goal of treatment is optimal management, analogous to the approach taken to other chronic diseases such as diabetes mellitus or rheumatoid arthritis. The aim of this chapter is to discuss several general management issues and to suggest an integrated overview of MS care.

Revealing the Diagnosis

On the basis of the stratified approach presented in Chapter 5, *Diagnosis and Differential Diagnosis*, most patients with neurological symptoms suggestive of MS may be confidently divided into groups in which:

- MS appears quite unlikely
- MS cannot be included or excluded on available evidence
- MS seems very probable.

In each of these instances, the diagnostic formulation should be communicated in a direct, but sympathetic, way.

If MS is very unlikely, the patient should be told so frankly, along with a discussion of alternative diagnoses and a suggested plan for appropriate continued care and follow-up. In the particular case in which there is no evidence for a primary neurological disease (eg, benign paresthesias, chronic fatigue syndrome, somatization disorder), firmness, tact, and diplomacy are required. Patients whose complaints appear to be functional, or without basis in definite neurological disease, can be among the most challenging in medicine. Several excellent, practical guides to the management of somatization and related disorders are available.[25,26,244,281,346] Keys to treating these persons are to establish a trusting relationship with one physician who will monitor the patient, perform or limit investigations and consultations appropriately, modify maladaptive behavior and thought patterns, encourage restoration of function, diagnose and treat psychiatric comorbidity, and confront when necessary. Often the time-constrained neurologist is not the ideal caregiver in these circumstances, and referral to a skilled primary care practitioner or psychiatrist is preferred, provided that such referral is made in a way that does not leave the patient with a sense of abandonment or stigmatization.

If MS cannot be included or excluded with confidence, further workup, regular follow-up visits, and indicated consultations should be pursued. In this instance, the patient should be helped to tolerate diagnostic uncertainty. All patients will be helped by assurances that support will be provided during their workup, including treatment of symptoms and regular updates, until the definitive diagnosis and treatment plan may be instituted.

When the diagnosis of MS is established, several key issues should be discussed with the patient (Table 8.1). Dr. Labe Scheinberg,[334] one of the pioneers of modern MS management, remarks:

There is a need for the neurologist to play a very active role in the early diagnostic revelations and education of the patient and family and not to relegate these matters to social workers, nurse clinicians, or even a chapter volunteer... This sort

**TABLE 8.1 — REVEALING THE DIAGNOSIS:
WHAT IS WRONG? WHAT CAN
WE DO ABOUT IT?**

- *Diagnosis:* Directly tell the patient that multiple sclerosis (MS) is established or highly likely. Since no test or finding is absolutely pathognomonic, some degree of uncertainty and need for periodic diagnostic review will carry into the future, especially if the patient has findings or a disease course that is atypical
- *Education:* Explain key features of the disease, such as the tendency for relapses, usually followed by substantial recovery in most cases. Counter excessive, misguided pessimism that many patients have based on chance encounters with exceptionally severe MS in acquaintances or through the media (see Chapter 8, *Prognosis and Management*)
- *Treatment options:* Explain that while there is no cure for MS, reasonably effective treatment exists for relapses, symptoms, and underlying disease course. Often patient-information packets and videos describing approved disease-modifying medications can be introduced at this point as a basis for subsequent counseling and decisions regarding management
- *Resources:* Provide telephone, e-mail, or other means of contact regarding new symptoms or questions. Tell patients of available self-help and other relevant sources of aid and information (see Chapter 9, *Resources*), such as those that may be obtained from the National Multiple Sclerosis Society. Every patient should be encouraged to become a member of the National Multiple Sclerosis Society
- *Partnership:* Encourage the patient and significant other(s) to join with the physician and other health care members as a unified team, working together to fight MS and make the best of a difficult situation

8

of thing I see as very important. The neurologist should take the responsibility of telling the patient and talking to the patient, educating the patient. You cannot relegate this to someone else.

In a larger sense, revealing the diagnosis implies going beyond merely providing a name for the patient's disease. Additionally, the patient should be given some insight into the implications of the diagnosis of MS and, in a preliminary way, told what the plan of management will be. By the time testing has been completed, most patients have anticipated MS or something like it; also, most patients will express relief that a definite cause exists to account for their symptoms. However, at some level all patients also experience a degree of emotional shock when the words "multiple sclerosis" are finally, definitely pronounced and they realize that this condition will be with them for the rest of their life.

The primary need of the patient at this point is calm reassurance that "life is not over," that many prior patients have been happy and successful despite their MS, and that support will be given to help the patient learn to live satisfactorily with MS. Although the key points in Table 8.1 should be made in a reassuring way and the patient's questions answered, lengthy discussions beyond the patient's ability to absorb and retain in a period of emotional stress should be avoided. Often investing time in a later clinic visit set aside to review the diagnosis and answer a list of questions provided by the patient is worthwhile and will bear substantial dividends in terms of a stable and compliant patient. Local chapters of the National Multiple Sclerosis Society often provide programs *specifically* designed to provide information and peer support for persons *recently* diagnosed with MS.

Prognosis

A schematic diagram depicting the natural history of an average or typical patient with MS is shown in Figure 8.1. While instructive as an overview of the

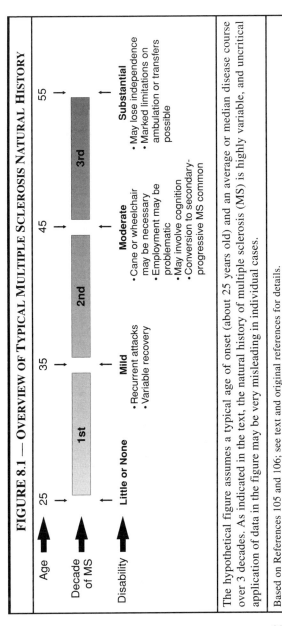

FIGURE 8.1 — OVERVIEW OF TYPICAL MULTIPLE SCLEROSIS NATURAL HISTORY

Age	25	35	45	55
Decade of MS	1st	2nd	3rd	
Disability	Little or None	Mild	Moderate	Substantial

Little or None

Mild
• Recurrent attacks
• Variable recovery

Moderate
• Cane or wheelchair may be necessary
• Employment may be problematic
• May involve cognition
• Conversion to secondary-progressive MS common

Substantial
• May lose independence
• Marked limitations on ambulation or transfers possible

The hypothetical figure assumes a typical age of onset (about 25 years old) and an average or median disease course over 3 decades. As indicated in the text, the natural history of multiple sclerosis (MS) is highly variable, and uncritical application of data in the figure may be very misleading in individual cases.

Based on References 105 and 106; see text and original references for details.

227

most typical course of MS, this figure *may be very misleading* if uncritically applied because of:

- *Individual variability.* MS outcomes vary widely among individual patients, from acutely fatal (Marburg variant) to virtually asymptomatic (benign variant). For many patients, the outlook may be quite favorable; for example, in the population-based natural history study from London, Ontario, almost 20% of the cohort of MS patients followed for 25 years had minimal, nonincapacitating disability (Disability Status Scale [DSS] <3.0).[105] Also, in Kurtzke's study[207] of patients with severe MS at onset, over 40% had improved neurological function at 10 years of follow-up.

- *Disease heterogeneity.* As indicated in Chapter 3, *Immunology, Pathogenesis, and Etiology*, there are hints from pathological and immunological investigations that indicate that different subsets of MS patients may have different pathophysiologies; in this sense, MS may not be one disease. Patients with primary-progressive MS (PPMS), for example, generally have a prognosis that is worse than that of the typical relapsing-remitting MS (RRMS) patient depicted in Figure 8.1.

- *Modification of natural history.* It is hoped that the application of disease-modifying treatments will favorably alter the relentless natural history course shown in Figure 8.1; it is also hoped that improved symptomatic treatment will lessen the impact of MS.

Several clinical features with prognostic value at onset or during the early course of MS have been identified, including such favorable variables as female sex, relapsing-remitting course, complete recovery after first attack, long interval between attacks, early age, sensory rather than motor symptoms, and MRI studies that are normal or show minimal disease.[105,106] While these early indicators have been carefully validated for *populations* of patients, unfortunately variation within populations is such that *an individual's* future clinical course cannot be predicted with high precision or confidence at onset. At best, a predominance of either favorable or unfavorable features at presentation allow an educated guess that the tempo of a patient's MS is likely to be slower or accelerated in comparison with the average or median course depicted in Figure 8.1. Accordingly, this relative, qualified projection can be useful in terms of individual counseling and management, eg, in identifying those patients in whom workup and treatment are particularly urgent. Recently, Scott and colleagues[343] have prospectively confirmed that short-term prognosis may be predicted from onset on the basis of specific indicators (Tables 8.2 and 8.3); also, the clinical analysis of risk may be complemented with prospectively validated MRI prognostic features at onset (Chapter 4, *Neuroimaging*).

In contrast to the qualified prognostic guess that may be made for a patient at onset or early in the disease course, once the patient has an *established* disease course, eg, after 5 years of MS, this course is a very robust prognostic indicator of long-term outcome on an individual level.[207] Thus, Kurtzke and associates found that only 11% of patients with mild disability at 5 years from diagnosis developed severe disability at 15 years. Even this reliable "5-year rule of Kurtzke" has exceptions, however. A case from personal practice comes to mind in which 20 years since diagnosis had passed without further attacks or disability; despite assurance of a benign course, a substantial attack occurred at 21 years! Exceptions such as this case do not invalidate useful prognostic rules; they

TABLE 8.2 — PREDICTION OF SHORT-TERM* MS PROGNOSIS: DELINEATION OF RISK FACTORS

Prognostic Risk Factor	Definition of Positive Risk
Age at onset	>40 years of age
Symptoms at onset	Motor alone or sensory plus motor
MRI status	Suggestive of definite MS ($\geq$4 typical lesions $\geq$3 mm on T2-weighted head study)
Interval between first and second attacks[†]	<2.5 years
Attack frequency in first 2 years[†]	>2 attacks
Completeness of recovery from initial attack	Poor (EDSS >2 after attack)

Abbreviations: EDSS, expanded disability status scale; MS, multiple sclerosis; MRI, magnetic resonance imaging.

* Short-term applies to approximately 3 years follow-up.
† Technically, the interval between attacks and attack frequency is unknown at onset. Nonetheless, when first seen in the clinic, many patients can relate a history of prior symptoms which likely represent genuine attacks; also, many patients will experience an additional attack shortly after initial evaluation. Thus in practice, the interval between first and second attacks and attack frequency in the first 2 years usually may be assessed early in the disease course and therefore may meaningfully contribute to prognostication for the succeeding 3- to 5-year period.

Adapted from Reference 343.

TABLE 8.3 — PREDICTION OF SHORT-TERM MS PROGNOSIS: SCORING OF RISK FACTORS FROM TABLE 8.2 AND ASSIGNMENT OF RISK TO PROGNOSTIC GROUPS

MS Prognostic Group*	Positive Risk Factors[†]	Initial EDSS[‡]	Final EDSS[§]	Time to Worsening (Months)[¶]
Low-risk group	0-1	1.1	1.3	60.8
Medium-risk group	2-3	1.3	1.8	83.5
High-risk group	4-6	1.4	3.7	33.9

Abbreviations: EDSS, expanded disability status scale; MS, multiple sclerosis.

Important qualifications and methodological considerations apply; for example, the low-risk group had only one patient, and risk factors were not entirely independent. Also, approximately 70% of patients were treated with disease modifying medications, and thus the cohort does not represent a pure natural history study. Despite these qualifications, the population under consideration is representative of that in most clinical practices and does serve as a useful guide to prognostication. The original study should be consulted for a complete explanation of these and other issues.

* In this study, patients were assigned to low-, medium-, and high-risk MS prognostic groups on the basis of the total number of positive factors identified (Table 8.2). The disease courses of these groups were compared over an average follow-up of 3 years in terms of change in disability score and estimated time to worsen one EDSS step.

† From Table 8.2.

‡ EDSS score (0 = no disability and 10 = death from MS) at diagnosis of clinically definite MS.

§ Mean EDSS at final evaluation, approximately 3 years follow-up.

¶ Average time to worsening of MS by 1.0 point on the EDSS scale, estimated from Kaplan-Meier survival analysis.

Adapted from Reference 343.

8

merely indicate that prognosis should be given with appropriate caution.

General Management Issues

■ Heat, Fever, Infection

Physiological investigations have shown that demyelinated fibers are exquisitely susceptible to minor elevations of temperature or mild acidosis.[160,392] The clinical implication of this finding is that exposure to heat (hot tubs, sauna, "baking in the sun"), fever (even 1° to 2°C), and infection should be avoided if possible and dealt with promptly when present. In this regard, several studies have documented the propensity of MS relapses to occur shortly after minor upper respiratory infections.[274,347] An illustrative MS case was that of a university neuroscientist, admitted in coma after a urinary tract infection and fever of 39°C; upon treatment with antibiotics, antipyretics, and cooling blankets, he promptly regained consciousness and subjected his intern to a lecture on the latest research findings from the laboratory. Often patients with severe brain stem attacks and impending respiratory and bulbar failure can be rescued by simply insisting on the vigorous application of cooling measures, such as maximal air conditioning and the use of a room fan to adequately circulate air. Although the classical teaching is that treatment of infection should be monitored by following the patient's temperature curve, MS patients constitute an important exception where the *treatment of fever itself is imperative and may dramatically improve the patient's neurological functioning.*

■ Anesthesia and Surgery

Early studies suggested that anesthesia and surgery constituted risk factors for attacks or deterioration of MS. However, more recent reports have called this hypothesis into question and indicate that the risk

232

from anesthesia or surgery, if present, is relatively small and therefore worth taking in MS patients in whom there is a strong indication for an operation. For example, Ridley and Schapira[309] reported on 40 MS patients who had no exacerbations in the month postsurgery. Also, Sibley and colleagues[348] found that the exacerbation rate in 125 MS patients studied prospectively was not increased in the 6-month period postsurgery in comparison with the 6-month period prior to surgery. Several reports suggest that MS patients are particularly susceptible to worsening after neurosurgical procedures, although this finding is controversial, and it is clear that appropriately selected MS patients have derived benefit from spinal decompression, ablative or microvascular treatment for trigeminal neuralgia, or deep brain stimulation and microlesional procedures for movement disorders. Perhaps a reasonable resolution of the controversial role of anesthesia and surgery in MS is to enthusiastically support intervention in patients when a clear and compelling indication exists ("as if the patient does not have MS"), but to advise caution and restraint for cosmetic or highly elective surgery. Most MS patients appear to tolerate anesthesia well,[3] although intrathecal or spinal anesthetics are generally avoided, given the proximity of cerebrospinal fluid (CSF) to vulnerable sites of demyelination. Epidural anesthetics, eg, for obstetrics, are well tolerated by MS patients.

■ **Contraception and Pregnancy**

In MS the endocrine and immune systems appear to be joined in a complex web whose interactions and significance are only partially understood.[84] For example, during pregnancy the relative risk of exacerbation falls precipitously, only to rebound in the postpartum period (Figure 8.2). That the magnitude of decline in relapse rate (RR) observed during pregnancy exceeds the reduction in RR achieved with approved

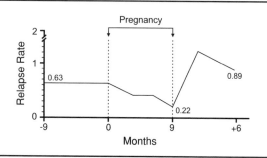
disease-modifying medications has not escaped the notice of investigators. Intuitively, this finding makes sense, since the activity of a putative autoimmune disease such as MS would be expected to decline during pregnancy, a time of relative immunosuppression that is protective for the developing fetus. Because of these findings, intensive investigation of the effect of hormones such as estrogen and progesterone on MS has been undertaken, both at the level of basic science[81,193] and exploratory clinical trials. At this stage in our knowledge, it appears that the influence of pregnancy on MS, while profound, is complex and not simply mediated through the action of one or two hormones.

What are the clinical implications of these findings for patients, many of whom are young women of childbearing age?

- The effect of oral contraceptives on the course of MS is controversial. Currently, there does not appear to be either a major beneficial or a deleterious effect of oral contraceptives on MS, and thus their use is a matter of personal choice to be made by the patient after discussion with her gynecologist. An exception to this statement might be the very rare MS patient in whom attacks of MS are clearly linked to menses[84]; in such cases specific hormonal therapy may be of use and should be discussed with the patient's gynecologist.

- Most women with MS experience a normal pregnancy, delivery, and puerperium. As depicted in Figure 8.2, the relative risk of attack falls during pregnancy and rises after pregnancy, effects which largely cancel each other out as statistical probabilities. Therefore, the decision to become pregnant and the obstetrical conduct of pregnancy may usually be made independently of MS. During delivery, all forms of anesthetics, including epidural analgesia, may be given, although intrathecal (spinal) anesthesia is traditionally avoided (as noted).

- Rare exceptions to the guidelines (listed above) include patients in whom a relative recommendation against pregnancy or parenthood should be considered because of incapacitating physical or emotional disability or other severe comorbidity. Fortunately, such circumstances are rare, and the majority of women with MS should be encouraged to have children, if that is their wish. On the other hand, given the possibility or probability of at least moderate disability over the course of MS in 20 to 30 years, some patients may choose to avoid or limit their responsibilities for child rearing. Quite obviously, in the context of MS, the decision to have or not have children is primarily a personal and not a medical one; nevertheless, factual information and discussions provided by the physician may significantly help the patient and her spouse with this question.

- Most authorities and official regulations indicate that the first-line disease-modifying treatments (Avonex, Betaseron, Copaxone, Rebif) are contraindicated during pregnancy and breastfeeding. Although the risk of teratogenicity does not appear to be substantial with these agents on current evidence, their use cannot be recommended in a patient who is or is attempting to become pregnant. Ideally, disease-modifying treatments should be discontinued at least 30 to 60 days prior to anticipated conception; if a woman on treatment becomes pregnant, the medication should be discontinued as soon as pregnancy is known. (Parenthetically, similar consideration would apply to most medications given for symptomatic treatment of MS, such as corticosteroids or antifatigue treatments. In each instance, the relative risks and benefits of medication during conception and pregnancy should be discussed with the pharmacist, obstetrician, and patient.) There is no firm evidence concerning the effect of disease-modifying treatments on sperm. Also, to date, there is no evidence of a rebound or exaggerated risk of MS activity immediately after cessation of disease-modifying treatment; in other words, statistically it appears that the patient's risk of attack when treatment stops merely reverts to the pretreatment risk, but does not overshoot this risk. In fact, if the medications are stopped during the relatively protected period of pregnancy, the allover risk of MS flare remains low.
- Since the postpartum period is one of increased risk for MS activity, it is generally recommended that disease-modifying treatment be reinstituted immediately after delivery and that the child be nursed with formula. There is anecdotal evidence that measures to reduce postpartum

stress and sleep deprivation have a favorable influence on MS, and it would seem prudent to recommend such measures insofar as possible and consistent with the patient's circumstances.

- In contrast to first-line agents, cytotoxic treatments such as mitoxantrone have demonstrated high teratogenic potential and thus are absolutely contraindicated during conception, pregnancy, and breast-feeding. Less certain are the long-term consequences of such treatment on mutagenesis and fertility; available animal data and limited human experience suggest these risks may be low but not insignificant. Thus the decisions to initiate cytotoxic treatment and to have children after cytotoxic treatment should only be made after discussion of these risks and uncertainties with the patient.

- The risk of MS in the offspring of an index case is in the order of 1% to 2%, a reassuring figure for most patients.

- Taken together, the statistics noted are generally favorable with regard to pregnancy and parenthood for patients with MS, and a positive outlook may be endorsed for these happy and life-affirming events. Nevertheless, experienced neurologists can recall individual instances in which a devastating attack occurred in the postpartum period or severe MS developed in a patient's child. Thus the risks noted, while statistically small, are potentially large in terms of impact on emotional and physical well-being and should always be discussed frankly with each patient of childbearing age.

■ Childhood Multiple Sclerosis

In most series, MS onset before age 10 is very rare (estimated 0.2% of MS cases), and MS at age 15 or less is uncommon (3% to 4% of MS cases).[29,229, 280,324]

In theory, the differential diagnosis of MS in childhood includes all the diseases discussed in Chapter 5, *Diagnosis and Differential Diagnosis*. Consideration of leukodystrophy or other degenerative disease is particularly relevant when there is a family history of neurological disease or when the child has a syndrome of insidious onset and steady progression. Nevertheless, in practice most childhood cases have an acute or subacute presentation, often in the setting of a febrile illness, and the most important differential diagnostic consideration is acute disseminated encephalomyelitis (ADEM).[217] Although none of these findings are absolutely discriminating between the two diseases, features that favor ADEM over MS include:

- Young age
- High fever
- Headache
- Drowsiness
- Seizures
- Bilateral simultaneous optic neuritis
- High CSF cell count
- Lack of CSF oligoclonal bands and IgG synthesis
- Aggressive MRI with all lesions at the same stage of activity or with hemorrhagic lesions
- Severe myelopathy with areflexia.

By contrast, an older patient with an absence of systemic or toxic features and with a typical CSF and MRI profile is more likely to develop MS. In essence, the condition in such patients may be thought of as typical MS with an onset in childhood; that is, there does not appear to be a distinctive syndrome of juvenile MS.

Since MS with childhood onset is unusual, there are no large, controlled studies to guide management. Certainly, the initial attack is usually treated with corticosteroids. Often a period of observation is helpful in making the distinction between ADEM and MS. In typical ADEM, the disease is monophasic, and no new clinical attacks or MRI changes should be apparent on reassessment during the 12- to 18-month period after the acute illness. Treatment of childhood MS with disease-modifying medications is problematic, since the pivotal phase 3 studies leading to FDA approval were all performed in adults. Nonetheless, if the diagnosis of definite, active MS is established, most neurologists recommend disease-modifying treatment. Since the long-term consequences of treating children with a normal component of their immune system, ie, human interferon, are unknown, a case could be made for initiating treatment with Copaxone, although favorable results and apparent safety have been reported in individual cases treated with interferon.[2]

■ **Vaccination**

Early vaccines containing neural tissue often evoked severe neurological reactions, and anecdotal reports have noted MS flares after virtually every vaccine. On the basis of these findings, in past decades many authorities have cautioned against vaccination in MS. Recently, however, large controlled trials have provided considerable evidence that vaccination is safe for patients with MS. In fact, a positive benefit has been demonstrated in some cases. For example, de Keyser and associates[94] demonstrated that the rate of MS exacerbation was 33% 6 weeks after influenza infection; in contrast, the risk of relapse was only 6% after influenza immunization. Also, BCG vaccine has been shown to have a benefit in a pilot study of MS activity monitored by MRI.[310]

Recently, a large study indicated no risk of short-term relapse in MS after common vaccines such as influenza, tetanus, and hepatitis B,[79] while a second large study showed no association between prior hepatitis B vaccination and the development of MS.[17] Actually, in the study of Confavreux and colleagues,[79] most vaccinations were associated with a lowered risk of MS relapse, although this effect did not achieve statistical significance. While several investigators have questioned specific findings of these reports on methodological grounds, a general consensus has emerged that vaccination is safe in MS and should be recommended when there are compelling indications.[105,122] A prudent exception would be to defer vaccination during an exacerbation or period of very active disease. Table 8.4 provides a summary of published immunization schedules for normal adults and for MS patients; original reports should be consulted for details and discussion of controversial points. Flachenecker and associates[122] in particular provide a comprehensive review of the literature relating each vaccine to MS and to vaccination during disease-modifying treatment. Additionally, Avery[19] provides a cogent discussion of vaccination in immunocompromised adults.

■ Exercise and Diet

Numerous studies have affirmed the general medical benefits of exercise, while implicating lack of exercise as a contributory factor in serious health problems such as obesity, hypertension, and coronary artery disease. With regard to MS, controlled studies have confirmed the benefit of aerobic exercise on measures of physical, emotional, and social well-being.[286] Obviously, general medical clearance should be obtained before starting vigorous activity, and supervision of the patient should continue throughout the exercise program. Patients should be encouraged to engage in any physical activity they enjoy, subject only to prohibitions against overheating (counter with fans, loose clothing), dehydration (avoid with frequent cold fluids), exhaustion (eg, "feel worse the next day"), and unsafe conditions (eg, potential for falls). Moderate elevations of body temperature during active exercise may be associated with transient minor symptoms such

240

as paresthesias or visual blurring; so far as is known, such symptoms have no lasting negative effects, and most neurologists do not consider them a contraindication to exercise, especially when the latter is known to be beneficial. Many MS patients benefit from swimming exercises (provided the pool is not too hot, ie, water should be <82°C), yoga, Tai-Chi, stretching exercises, ergometric exercises primarily using the upper extremities, and the like. Often exercise classes or programs designed specifically for persons with disabilities are available through local health clubs or sports medicine facilities. At times, consultation with a recreation therapist, sports medicine physician, or physiatrist may help in formulating an exercise prescription to meet an individual's needs. Keys to compliance with a long-term exercise program are activities that the patient enjoys, socialization, positive reenforcement, a regular schedule of planned exercises, and the requirement for at least nominal fees or other demonstrations of personal commitment.

Despite considerable enthusiasm, there is no convincing objective scientific evidence that any of the many diets proposed has a positive effect on the course of MS.[295] Swank[50] has popularized a low-fat diet based on the rationale that populations with minimal animal fat intake, such as Asians, have a low incidence of MS. Although success of this diet has been claimed in long-term studies, these findings have been questioned in terms of methodological grounds, such inappropriate controls and incomplete follow-up. Many of the diets proposed for MS, eg, the low-fat regimens, appear benign and may favorably influence general health, provided that they are not burdensome personally or financially and do not produce severe nutritional imbalance.

TABLE 8.4 — IMMUNIZATION RECOMMENDATIONS FOR MS PATIENTS*

Patient Group	Recommended Immunization Schedule[††]									Ref
	Influenza	Pneumo-coccal	Hep B	Tetanus-Diphtheria	Polio	Varicella	Hep A	MMR		
Normal adults	If at risk, annual immuni-zation	If at risk, revaccinate at 6 years, sche-dule uncertain thereafter	If at risk, every 10 years	Boosters	Childhood	Childhood	If at risk, single series	Childhood		1
Demonstrated safety in MS patients[§]	+++	?	+++	+ Tetanus ++ Diptheria	+	?	?	+ Measles ? Mumps + Rubella		2
MS, normal otherwise	As per routine adult indications and schedules above, assuming patient is not in the midst of an active flare or acutely immunosuppressed									2
MS, receiving disease-modifying treatment	Presumably recommendations are identical to those for untreated healthy MS adults, although there are no large studies directly addressing this issue; by inferences based on experience with other patients on immuno-modulating (eg, interferon) or intermittent immunosuppressive (eg, mitoxantrone) therapy, administration of vaccines such as Hep B and influenza appear to be safe and effective. In the absence of controlled investiga-tions of vaccinations during disease-modifying treatment in MS, clinical judgment as to relative risks and benefits in each patient should be applied.									2

MS, continuous immunosuppression or severe disabilitation	Immunization is surprisingly safe and effective in immunosuppressed patients, although all live vaccines (varicella and MMR) are contraindicated. Generally, influenza vaccine is recommended yearly, pneumococcal vaccine possibly ≥6 years, and tetanus-diptheria boosters every 10 years. Other vaccines should be given to patients at high risk or in special circumstances. See Avery[19] for details.

Abbreviations: Hep B, hepatitis B; Hep A, hepatitis A; MMR, measles, mumps, rubella; MS, multiple sclerosis.

* Based on current consensus of most authorities and available results; text and original sources should be consulted with regard to controversies and ongoing research.

† *At Risk:* See Gardner and Peter[129] or consult with an infectious diseases expert for definition of risk and for special cases. The recommendations of Gardner and Peter[129] are based on those of the Advisory Committee on Immunization Practices and the American College of Physicians. In general, residents of long-term care facilities, the elderly, and patients with chronic debilitating cardiopulmonary, renal, diabetic, or similar diseases are considered at risk for influenza and pneumococcus. Occupational or personal exposure, eg, health care workers, travelers, susceptible family members of immunocompromised patients, may be at special risk, especially to Hep B. "Childhood" designation assumes that the adult had recommended immunizations in childhood; see Garder and Peter[129] for schedules in unimmunized adults and Avery[19] for adults who must be reimmunized because of immunodeficiency.

‡ *Hep A,* inactivated virus; *Hep B,* viral protein expressed by recombinant DNA methods; *Influenza,* inactivated virus components; *MMR,* life attenuated virus; *Pneumococcal,* capsid polysaccharides components; *Polio,* inactivated virus; *Tetanus and Diptheria,* inactivated bacterial toxins; *Varicella,* live attenuated virus.

§ ? = no adequate controlled studies; + = safe in small controlled studies; ++ = safe in several retrospective surveys; +++ = safe in prospective, placebo and double-blind studies.

[1]Gardner and Peter, 2001 (Reference 129); [2]Flachenecker et al, 2001 (Reference 122); [3]Avery, 2001 (Reference 19).

■ Alternative and Complementary Medicine

Bowling[42] defines complementary and alternative medicine (CAM) as "medical approaches, such as acupuncture or herbal medicine, that are not typical components of conventional medicine." By definition, then, evaluation of CAM would seem problematic for conventional practitioners. Physicians' attitudes range from enthusiasm and active recommendation for CAM (on the basis of hope and benefits provided by these treatments) to agnosticism and a call for further research (given surveys showing that two thirds of MS patients have taken at least one CAM treatment) and, finally, to hostility for CAM, since most claims are unproven and treatment has been harmful in some instances. The following recommendations would seem prudent regarding CAM and MS:

- Practitioners who advocate or sanction CAM treatment should be knowledgeable with regard to the therapy and should be prepared to assume responsibility for and treatment of any adverse consequences of therapy.
- Physicians should be aware of CAM treatments that may adversely affect MS (Table 8.5).
- Patients should be apprised of telltale signs indicating unreliable forms of CAM, including heavy reliance on testimonials, extraordinary claims of effectiveness ("too good to be true"), antagonism to conventional medicine, promotion of conspiracy theories, and lack of reliable, objective information concerning safety and effectiveness.[42]

Bowling[42] and Polman and colleagues[295] provide detailed and informative evaluations of individual CAM treatments for MS.

TABLE 8.5 — COMPLEMENTARY AND ALTERNATIVE MEDICAL TREATMENTS THAT MAY ADVERSELY AFFECT MS*

- Herbs that may stimulate the immune system:[†]
  - Alfalfa
  - Echinacea
  - Garlic
  - Ginseng
  - Licorice
  - Mistletoe
  - Shiitake mushroom
  - Stinging nettle
  - Woody night-shade stem
- Herbs that may interact with corticosteroids:[‡]
  - Ginseng
  - Ephedra
  - Licorice
  - Senna
- Herbs that may interact with antidepressant medications:[§]
  - St. John's wort
  - Belladonna
  - Henbane
  - Mistletoe
  - Scopolia

---

* Only the most commonly administered treatments are listed; see Bowling[42] for comprehensive listing, in-depth reviews, and original citations.

† Caution is based on the supposition that multiple sclerosis is an autoimmune disease and that further stimulation of the immune system will increase multiple sclerosis activity.

‡ These herbs may worsen the side effects or increase the potency of corticosteroids.

§ These herbs should be avoided with either tricyclic or selective serotonin reuptake inhibitor antidepressants.

Table based on Reference 42.

■ Psychosocial Issues and Disability

It is not surprising that a chronic disorder that eventually may result in significant physical and mental disability often has a negative impact on a patient's interactions with family, work, and society. In the worst case, a patient may feel that their life is not worth living. Thus epidemiological surveys have shown that MS is one of the medical disorders that are associated with an increased risk of suicide, a risk that primarily depends on depression and the plight of persons severely disabled by neurological disease. Specifically, the risk of suicide in MS patients is approximately 2.35 times that in normals in relative terms and 8/1000 persons in absolute terms.[155]

Surprisingly, epidemiological analysis of other severely disabling diseases, such as amyotrophic lateral sclerosis, stroke, cancer, rheumatoid arthritis, ankylosing spondylitis, and viral liver disease, reveals an average risk of suicide, probably because these conditions usually are not associated with prominent mental disorder.[155] These statistics indicate the need for vigorous surveillance and treatment of depression in all patients with MS (Chapter 7, *Symptomatic Treatment*).

In addition to the risk engendered by depression, it is also thought that suicide risk in MS patients may be exacerbated by the communicated perception of society and even caretakers that the patient's quality of life is "unacceptable" or a "burden." By contrast, the same epidemiological investigations have shown that medical conditions such as pregnancy and puerperium, although sometimes associated with depression and even psychosis, are characterized by a *decreased risk of suicide* relative to the normal population.[155] Evidently, when persons have a positive goal to live for, such as being a parent, suicide risk is greatly diminished. Against the negative perception of quality of life in MS (or even the assumption that individual lives can be judged as being more or less worthy), a recent publication provides a collection of 31 biographies of remarkable persons who have overcome the adversity of MS and made inspiring contributions to society (*Incidental Heros: Disabling the Myths About Multiple Sclerosis*).[145]

A number of practical guides to help patients with psychosocial issues and disability are listed in Chapter 9, *Resources*. A volume that is particularly useful to both patients and physicians is *Multiple Sclerosis: Your Legal Rights* by Lanny Perkins and Sara Perkins.[285] Local chapters of the National Multiple Sclerosis Society also provide useful guidance and information in this regard.

A particularly vexing issue for patients and physicians is that of employment and disability benefits. At onset, almost all persons with MS are able to work and thus should be encouraged to participate in gainful and satisfying employment. Nevertheless, as decades pass, MS often produces constraints on employment; one estimate is that 15 years postdiagnosis, only 15% of MS patients are working.[403] It is hoped that this dismal statistic may be improved with better MS treatment, more enlightened societal attitudes, and improved support for persons with MS.

Often the ability of persons with MS to work is seen in black and white terms, ie, comparing early disease, when work is unrestricted, and advanced disease, when any work is impossible. The real difficulty for patients and physicians usually occurs in the intermediate case, the gray zone of disability, when MS produces significant limitations but does not preclude work altogether and does not qualify the patient for permanent disability benefits. Solutions are not easy to come by but may include reduced hours or duties, alterations of the work conditions, within-company transfers, a planned leave of absence, short-term disability, or consideration of alternative employment.

247

Often a vocational counselor can assist patients and employers to pursue these options in a creative and mutually beneficial, rather than antagonistic, manner.

Historically, private and governmental disability benefit provisions were usually assembled piecemeal and are not entirely rational or helpful in the case of MS. For example, the Social Security Administration (SSA) considers benefits based on the concept of total disability, as defined by intricate criteria known as listing and grades.[285] Although these criteria are very formal, ultimately, systems such as SSA are administered by persons who usually are reasonable, of good will, and capable of applying existing rules with a degree of common sense and flexibility. Often several appeals must be made before disability status is granted.

The physician may be of help by providing documentation and medical reports to authorized disability reviewers. Often the physician serves a useful purpose by reminding lay adjudicators that MS is not a linear disease affecting one well-defined system (eg, as progressive renal failure is); instead, MS results from many lesions affecting several areas of the central nervous system simultaneously. Disability, then, in MS is commonly *multiplicative*, and several symptoms, which in themselves would not be incapacitating (eg, moderate fatigue, weakness, imbalance, cognitive change), are, in the aggregate, constitutive of profound disability.

■ Leisure and Recreation

Patients should be actively encouraged to pursue hobbies and leisure activities. These serve as useful outlets for frustration and buffer the patient from the negative impact of MS. Questions such as "What do you do for fun?" and "What are your hobbies?" should be part of the review of systems. Realism should be fostered, ie, recommending activities that appear to be within the patient's current or anticipated abilities.

■ Spirituality

Multiple sclerosis represents a major challenge to all aspects of a patient's existence. Many patients derive considerable solace from an organized religious, spiritual, or philosophical practice. Obviously, the physician's role is to provide health care, not spiritual guidance, but validating the patient's discussion of this area of life or encouraging the patient to follow up within his or her own tradition are legitimate and may help patients better cope with their disease. At times of crisis, referral to the appropriate hospital chaplain or pastor may be appreciated by the patient and family.

Hope and Optimism   8

A recent letter to the *Annals of Internal Medicine*[201] cites poet and former President of Czechoslovakia Vaclav Havel on the subject of hope:

Hope is an orientation of the spirit, an orientation of the heart; it is not the conviction that something will turn out well, but the certainty that something makes sense, regardless of how it turns out.

In the author's opinion, hope and optimism *make sense* when facing a chronic neurological disorder; these attitudes are practical weapons in the fight against MS, and their use by patients should be actively encouraged. Optimism can of course be overdone, and hope may be unrealistic. Reliance on quack cures and magical thinking should be gently resisted and corrected. MS is always unfortunate; even in the most benign instance of this disease, a patient must always live with uncertainty and the possibility of eventual attack or disability. Also, all patients normally experience grief, frustration, and discouragement at some point during the course of MS. These appropriate reactions should not be dismissed casually. As indicated, in addition to treatment and counseling provided by the physician, psychological and peer-group support may be of considerable help in allowing patients to express and constructively deal with these difficult emotions.

Recent psychological investigations have suggested that each person may have a relatively stable, invariant propensity to a given level of satisfaction and mood, an inherent "set point for happiness." Certainly, MS is no respecter of personality type, and MS affects those prone to either sunny or dark dispositions. Nevertheless, psychological investigations have also shown that a person's degree of optimism or pessimism may be significantly modified by cognitive therapy and other techniques. For these reasons, it is important for patient and practitioner to *cultivate* reasonable hope and optimism, to insist on the *habit* of seeing the proverbial glass as "half full, not half empty." Practical measures to encourage optimism and hope in the patient have been empirically studied in the context of chronic diseases, including MS (Table 8.6). While the interventions listed in the table are largely a matter of common sense and compassionate management, it is useful to explicitly consider the "little things" caregivers do that may have a large or even decisive impact on the patient.

In the sense indicated by Havel, successfully coping with this chronic neurological disease requires an active effort to maintain one's orientation in positive, hopeful ways. The advice given by many experienced patients with MS is to "hope for the best, while preparing for the possibility of the worst." All of us can reasonably expect that continued societal and scientific progress will lessen the burden of MS and decrease the suffering of our patients.

250

TABLE 8.6 — MEANS BY WHICH CARETAKERS MAY PROMOTE OPTIMISM AND HOPE IN MS PATIENTS

- Active reflection and self-awareness in caretaker ("resolve your own personal agenda," consider what attitudes are being conveyed overtly or unconsciously)[1]
- Affirm worth of patient (by showing respect, listening, touching, understanding)[1]
- Create a partnership with the patient (asymmetric but mutual: "the patient is central, not someone who is 'done unto' but someone who is negotiated with")[1]
- Address the totality of the patient as a unique individual (not "just another patient"; ask about specific concerns, hobbies, problems, family issues; consider the patient's specific psychological and cultural attributes)[1]
- Set most goals on a short-term basis (goals change as illness changes)[2]
- Emphasize effectiveness of certain interventions (disease-modifying treatment, corticosteroids, symptomatic treatment: "something can be done for your multiple sclerosis [MS]")[2]
- Note the generally good outlook for recovery after an exacerbation of MS, mention other positive prognostic factors[2]
- Concentrate on realistic, positive events[2]
- Acknowledge grief for lost functions and anxiety regarding unpredictability of MS; at the same time, help the patient to identify and visit a personal "*MS-Free Zone*," a psychological place that MS has not reached (eg, humor, music, religious faith, particular skill, or talent)[3]

[1]Adapted from Cutliff[88]; [2]Adapted from Carter[59]; [3]Adapted from National Multiple Sclerosis Society[253].

9   Resources

Numerous resources exist for both patients and physicians interested in multiple sclerosis (MS). A partial listing of useful sources of information is given below; a more extensive listing is beyond the scope of this handbook, but in most instances, these indicated sources will indicate where detailed or in-depth assistance is available.

Reference Texts

Several large, comprehensive volumes explore MS from basic science and clinical perspectives. Recent publications in this area include:

Burks JS, Johnson KP. *Multiple Sclerosis: Diagnosis, Medical Management, and Rehabilitation*[53]

Rudick RA, Goodkin DE. *Multiple Sclerosis Therapeutics*[323]

Compston A, Ebers G, Lassman H, McDonald I, Matthews B, Wekerle H. *McAlpine's Multiple Sclerosis*[75]

Cook SD. *Handbook of Multiple Sclerosis.*[80]

Paty DW, Ebers GC. *Multiple Sclerosis*[280]

Hawkins CP, Wolinksy JS. *Principles of Treatments in Multiple Sclerosis.*[157]

In addition, several recent reviews are very informative (Noseworthy et al[262]; Polman and Uitdehaag[294]; Wingerchuck[409])

Multiple Sclerosis Societies

Multiple sclerosis societies are the major institutions devoted to patient support and research into this disease. Listed below are contacts for the United States, Canada, United Kingdom, and the International Federation of MS Societies (with links to 34 national or regional associations). National multiple sclerosis societies provide information and assistance to patients, contacts to local chapters, bulletins on common symptoms and questions, help lines and support groups, research announcements, periodicals, links to other resources, and many other services.

National Multiple Sclerosis Society
733 Third Avenue
New York, New York
800-Fight MS (800-344-4867)
www.nmss.org

Multiple Sclerosis Society of Canada
250 Bloor Street East, Suite 1000
Toronto, Ontario M4W 3P9
416-922-6065
www.mssociety.ca

The MS National Center
372 Edgware Road
London NW2 6ND
020-843-80700
www.mssociety.org.uk

International Federation of Multiple Sclerosis Societies
10 Heddon Street
GB-London, W1R 7LJ
44-171-734-9120
www.ifmss.org.uk

Disease-Modifying Treatments

As indicated in Chapter 6, *Disease-Modifying Treatment*, Table 6.4, the manufacturers of approved disease-modifying treatments have established telephone and web support sites to provide information and patient instructions with regard to each medication. In addition, the sites provide general information, educational programs, and counseling concerning MS.

Demos Medical Publishing

One publisher, Demos Medical Publishing, has concentrated heavily on MS and provided many volumes of interest to patients and physicians. A complete listing of all Demos books relating to MS may be obtained at:

Demos Medical Publishing
386 Park Avenue South, Suite 201
New York, NY 10016
800-532-8663
www.demosmedpub.com

Several books may be of particular interest, such as:

Polman CH, Thompson AJ, Murray TJ, McDonald WI. *Multiple Sclerosis: The Guide to Treatment and Management.* 2001 (ISBN: 1-888799-54-4).

This volume is written by a panel of international experts who review conventional and alternative therapeutic claims in MS. A consensus opinion is given with regard to safety and efficacy of each agent, as well as original references for in-depth review. The style is clear and concise; remarkably, this authoritative reference simultaneously meets the needs of both lay and medical readers.

Holland NJ, Murray TJ, Reingold SC. *Multiple Sclerosis: A Guide for the Newly Diagnosed.* 1996 (ISBN: 1-888799-06-4).
The basic facts of MS are explained in lay terms; psychological insights, coping strategies, and symptom management are set out in helpful, practical terms.

Shapiro RT. *Symptom Management in Multiple Sclerosis.* 1998 (ISBN: 1-888799-22-6).
A comprehensive, multidisciplinary approach to MS symptoms is set out in practical, patient-oriented terms.

Kalb RC. *Multiple Sclerosis: A Guide for Families.* 1998 (ISBN: 1-888799-14-5).
Dr. Kalb and coauthors describe emotional issues, childbirth, caregivers, life and financial planning, general health, and other MS-related issues from the perspective of patient and family. Particularly useful are sections and appendices that detail publications, web sites, and contacts on numerous aspects of disability.

Bowling AC. *Alternative Medicine and Multiple Sclerosis.* 2001 (ISBN: 1-888799-52-8).
Dr. Bowling provides a very balanced, evidence-based discussion of herbal therapy, diets, exercise, acupuncture, homeopathy, chiropractic treatment,

and other alternative treatments. Side effects, costs, practical information, references, and contacts are provided for each modality.

Schwarz SP. *300 Tips for Making Life With Multiple Sclerosis Easier.* 1999 (ISBN: 1-888799-23-4).
The author is an engaging and practical person with MS, a self-described "problem-solver." In this and several similar publications, she provides very practical advice on managing MS in daily personal and family life.

Perkins L, Perkins S. *Multiple Sclerosis: Your Legal Rights.* 1999 (ISBN: 1-888799-31-5).
A comprehensive guide to disability law and other legal provisions relevant to MS is given; in addition, comprehensive advice on financial and personal planning for persons with MS is presented. The author has recommended or provided this volume for most of his patients.

9

Additionally, Demos has volumes specifically targeted for MS with regard to insurance, employment, rehabilitation, family life, progressive MS, pregnancy, caregiving, and other topics.

Internet Links for Multiple Sclerosis

In addition to web sites indicated, a number of sources provide comprehensive listing of links with relevance to MS, several of which are indicated below. Patients should be cautioned that this information is unregulated, and some of the entries may be misleading. Particular caution should be exercised with "copycat" organizations of questionable value or aims, whose name or web site is designed to mimic but subtly differ from established, legitimate institutions. In general, patients are well-advised to review any information they obtain with their physician, other health professionals, or authoritative sources such as the National Multiple Sclerosis Society.

Multiple Sclerosis Links
www.cybersourcegeneva.com/ms.html

Infosci's Home Page
www.infosci.org

Miscellaneous

Medic Alert Foundation
800-344-3226
www.medicaltert.org
This nonprofit foundation provides identification tags and medical information that can be accessed by a physician or emergency personnel.

ARC (formerly Association for Retarded Persons).
301-565-3842
www.thearc.org
ARC provides very helpful information and resources for all persons with disabilities.

NCIL (National Council on Independent Living)
703-525-3406
www.ncil.org
NCIL provides information and assistance for persons with disability.

Information for Handicapped Travelers
A booklet, available free from 800-424-8567 that provides information concerning travel agents and transportation for persons with disabilities. Other sources of information may be found in the book by Kalb, cited earlier.

ABLEDATA
800-227-0216
www.abledata.com
A database of assistive technology for persons with disabilities.

Eastern Paralyzed Veterans Association
718-803-EPVA
This organization will provide information and support to veterans and non-veterans with spinal cord injury or dysfunction.

Consortium of Multiple Sclerosis Centers
201-837-0727
www.mscare.org
The Consortium provides information about MS care and MS centers, including rehabilitative and experimental therapies.

International Multiple Sclerosis Support Foundation
www.msnews.org

Mayo Clinic Patient Information Site
www.mayo.edu
Search under "multiple sclerosis"; a general, patient-oriented overview of multiple sclerosis is provided, as well as links to subsidiary topics and the results of recent research.

National Institutes of Health
www.nlm.nih.gov/medlineplus/multiplesclerosis.html
The latest news and research on multiple sclerosis, general overviews, clinical trials, disease management, and links to other sites, including MedLine searches for recent articles on multiple sclerosis, are given.

Physician Consultation Resources

**National Multiple Sclerosis Society (NMSS)
Physician Consultation Service**
1-866-MS-TREAT or 800-678-7328
MD_info@nmss.org
Community physicians may contact the Professional
Resource Center of the National Multiple Sclerosis
Society by e-mail or telephone, and inquiries will be
passed to a member of the Medical Advisory Board
of the NMSS, who will reply directly.

REFERENCES

1. Adachi M, Hosoya T, Yamaguchi K, Kawanami T, Kato T. Diffusion- and T2-weighted MRI of the transverse pontine fibres in spinocerebellar degeneration. *Neuroradiology.* 2000;42:803-809.

2. Adams AB, Tyor WR, Holden KR. Interferon beta-1b and childhood multiple sclerosis. *Pediatr Neurol.* 1999;21:481-483.

3. Adams DC, Heyer EJ. Problems of anesthesia in patients with neuromuscular disease. *Anesthesiology Clin North Am.* 1997;15:673-689.

4. Akdeniz H, Irmak H, Anlar O, Demiroz AP. Central nervous system brucellosis: presentation, diagnosis and treatment. *J Infect.* 1998;36:297-301.

5. Akman-Demir G, Serdaroglu P, Tasci B. Clinical patterns of neurological involvement in Behcet's disease: evaluation of 200 patients. The Neuro-Behcet Study Group. *Brain.* 1999;122:2171-2182.

6. al Deeb SM, Yaqub BA, Bruyn GW, Biary NM. Acute transverse myelitis. A localized form of postinfectious encephalomyelitis. *Brain.* 1997;120:1115-1122.

7. Al-Fahad SA, Al-Araji AH. Neuro-Behcet's disease in Iraq: a study of 40 patients. *J Neurol Sci.* 1999;170:105-111.

8. Alanen A, Komu M, Penttinen M, Leino R. Magnetic resonance imaging and proton MR spectroscopy in Wilson's disease. *Br J Radiol.* 1999;72:749-756.

9. Alderson L, Fetell MR, Sisti M, Hochberg F, Cohen M, Louis DN. Sentinel lesions of primary CNS lymphoma. *J Neurol Neurosurg Psychiatry.* 1996;60:102-105.

10. Alexander E. Central nervous system disease in Sjogren's syndrome. New insights into immunopathogenesis. *Rheum Dis Clin North Am.* 1992;18:637-672.

11. Practice parameter: diagnosis of patients with nervous system Lyme borreliosis (Lyme disease)—summary statement. Report of the Quality Standards Subcommittee of the American Academy of Neurology. *Neurology.* 1996;46:881-882.

12. American Academy of Neurology 53rd annual meeting. May 5-11, 2001, Philadelphia Pennsylvania, USA. *Neurology.* 2001;56(8 suppl 3):A1-559.

13. Anderson M. Neurology of Whipple's disease. *J Neurol Neurosurg Psychiatry.* 2000;68:2-5.

14. Antiguedad A, Zarranz JJ. Eales disease involving central nervous system white matter (Spanish). *Neurologia.* 1994;9:307-310.

15. Armstrong C, Lewis T, D'Esposito M, Freundlich B. Eosinophilia-myalgia syndrome: selective cognitive impairment, longitudinal effects, and neuroimaging findings. *J Neurol Neurosurg Psychiatry.* 1997;63:633-641.

16. Arnold DL, Wolinsky JS, Matthews PM, Falini A. The use of magnetic resonance spectroscopy in the evaluation of the natural history of multiple sclerosis. *J Neurol Neurosurg Psychiatry.* 1998;64(suppl): S94-S101.

17. Ascherio A, Zhang SM, Hernan MA, et al. Hepatitis B vaccination and the risk of multiple sclerosis. *N Engl J Med.* 2001;344:327-332.

18. Atabay C, Erdem E, Kansu T, Eldem B. Eales disease with internuclear ophthalmoplegia. *Ann Ophthal.* 1992;24:267-269.

19. Avery RK. Immunizations in adult immunocompromised patients: which to use and which to avoid. *Cleve Clin J Med*. 2001;68:337-348.

20. Aylward EH, Roberts-Twillie JV, Barta PE, et al. Basal ganglia volumes and white matter hyperintensities in patients with bipolar disorder. *Am J Psychiatry*. 1994;151:687-693.

21. Bar-Or A, Oliveira EM, Anderson DE, Hafler DA. Molecular pathogenesis of multiple sclerosis. *J Neuroimmunol*. 1999;100:252-259.

22. Barkhof F, Filippi M, Miller DH, et al. Comparison of MRI criteria at first presentation to predict conversion to clinically definite multiple sclerosis. *Brain*. 1997;120:2059-2069.

23. Barnes M. Management of spasticity-pharmacological agents. In: Hawkins C, Wolinsky JS, eds. *Principles of Treatments in Multiple Sclerosis*. Oxford: Butterworth-Heinemann Medical; 2000:184-200.

24. Barnett M, Prosser J, Sutton I, et al. Paraneoplastic brain stem encephalitis in a woman with anti-Ma2 antibody. *J Neurol Neurosurg Psychiatry*. 2001;70:222-225.

25. Barsky AJ, Borus JF. Functional somatic syndromes. *Ann Intern Med*. 1999;130:910-921.

26. Barsky AJ. The patient with hypochondriasis. *N Engl J Med*. 2001;345:1395-1399.

27. Bartzokis G, Goldstein B, Hance IB, et al. The incidence of T2-weighted MR imaging signal abnormalities in the brain of cocaine-dependent patients is age-related and region-specific. *Am J Neuroradiol*. 1999;20:1628-1635.

28. Bashir K, Cai CY, Moore TA, Whitaker JN, Hadley MN. Surgery for cervical spinal cord compression in patients with multiple sclerosis. *Neurosurgery*. 2000;47:637-643.

29. Bauer HJ, Hanefeld. *Multiple Sclerosis: Its Impact from Childhood to Old Age*. London: Saunders, 1993.

30. Baum SG. *Mycoplasma pneumoniae* and atypical pneumonia. In: Mandell GL, Bennett JE, Dolin R, eds. *Principles and Practice of Infectious Diseases*. New York, NY: Churchill Livingstone; 2018-2027.

31. Beck RW, Cleary PA, Anderson MM, et al. A randomized, controlled trial of corticosteroids in the treatment of acute optic neuritis. The Optic Neuritis Study Group. *N Engl J Med*. 1992;326:581-588.

32. Beck RW, Cleary PA, Trobe JD, et al. The effect of corticosteroids for acute optic neuritis on the subsequent development of multiple sclerosis The Optic Neuritis Study Group. *N Engl J Med*. 1993;329:1764-1769.

33. Beck RW. The optic neuritis treatment trial: three-year follow-up results. *Arch Ophthalmol*. 1995;113:136-137.

34. Bemporad JA, Sze GS. MR imaging of spinal cord vascular malformations with an emphasis on the cervical spine. *Magn Reson Imaging Clin N Am*. 2000;8:581-596.

35. Berger JR, Tornatore C, Major EO, et al. Relapsing and remitting human immunodeficiency virus-associated leukoencephalomyelopathy. *Ann Neurol*. 1992;31:34-38.

36. Blackburn WD. Eosinophilia myalgia syndrome. *Semin Arthritis Rheum*. 1997;26:788-793.

37. Blinkenberg M, Jensen CV, Holm S, Paulson OB, Sorensen PS. A longitudinal study of cerebral glucose metabolism, MRI, and disability in patients with MS. *Neurology*. 1999;53:149-153.

38. Boehm CD, Cutting GR, Lachtermacher MB, Moser HW, Chong SS. Accurate DNA-based diagnostic and carrier testing for X-linked adrenoleukodystrophy. *Mol Genet Metab*. 1999;66:128-136.

39. Boers PM, Colebatch JG. Hashimoto's encephalopathy responding to plasmapheresis. *J Neurol Neurosurg Psychiatry*. 2001;70:132.

40. Bohnen NI, Parnell KJ, Harper CM. Reversible MRI findings in a patient with Hashimoto's encephalopathy. *Neurology*. 1997;49:246-247.

41. Bonkovsky HL, Barnard GF. Diagnosis of porphyric syndromes: a practical approach in the era of molecular biology. *Semin Liver Dis*. 1998;18:57-65.

42. Bowling AC. *Alternative Medicine and Multiple Sclerosis*. New York, NY: Demos Medical Publishing;2001.

43. Brady RO, Grabowski GA, Thadhani R. *Fabry disease: review and new perspectives*. SynerMed Communications; 2001.

44. Brecher K, Hochberg FH, Louis DN. Case report of unusual leukoencephalopathy preceding primary CNS lymphoma. *J Neurol Neurosurg Psychiatry*. 1998;65:917-920.

45. Brewer GJ, Fink JK, Hedera P. Diagnosis and treatment of Wilson's disease. *Sem Neurol*. 1999;19:261-270.

46. Brex PA, Miszkiel KA, O'Riordan JI, et al. Assessing the risk of early multiple sclerosis in patients with clinically isolated syndromes: the role of a follow-up MRI. *J Neurol Neurosurg Psychiatry*. 2001;70: 390-393.

47. Brey RL, Escalante A. Neurological manifestations of antiphospholipid antibody syndrome. *Lupus*. 1998;7(suppl 2):S67-S74.

48. Brillman J, Rohteram EB Jr, Valeriano JP, Scott TF, Thomas LC. The magnetic resonance image appearance of *Mycoplasma pneumoniae* encephalopathy. *J Neuroimag*. 1992;2:42-44.

49. Brisman R. Gamma knife radiosurgery for primary management for trigeminal neuralgia. *J Neurosurg*. 2000;93(suppl 3):159-161.

50. Britell CW, Burks JS. Alternative and complementary therapies. In: Burks JS, Johnson KP, eds. *Multiple Sclerosis: Diagnosis, Medical Management, and Rehabilitation*. New York, NY: Demos Medical Publishing;2000:491-504.

51. Broggi G, Ferroli P, Franzini A, Servello D, Dones I. Microvascular decompression for trigeminal neuralgia: comments on a series of 250 cases, including 10 patients with multiple sclerosis. *J Neurol Neurosurg Psychiatry*. 2000;68:59-64.

52. Bryant J, Clegg A, Milne R. Systematic review of immunomodulatory drugs for the treatment of people with multiple sclerosis: Is there good quality evidence on effectiveness and cost? *J Neurol Neurosurg Psychiatry*. 2001;70:574-579.

53. Burks JS, Johnson KP, eds. *Multiple Sclerosis: Diagnosis, Medical Management, and Rehabilitation*. New York, NY: Demos Medical Publishing;2000.

54. Burns WH, Burt RK. Hematopoietic stem cell transplantation. In: Rudick RA, Goodkin DE, eds. *Multiple Sclerosis Therapeutics*. London: Blackwell Science Inc; 1999:371-393.

55. Bushnell CD, Goldstein LB. Diagnostic testing for coagulopathies in patients with ischemic stroke. *Stroke*. 2000;31:3067-3078.

56. Calopa M, Marti T, Rubio F, Peres J. Magnetic resonance imaging and Cogan's syndrome (French). *Rev Neurol*. 1991;147:161-163.

57. Carmel R. Current concepts in cobalamin deficiency. *Ann Rev Med*. 2000;51:357-375.

10

58. Carrigan DR, Harrington D, Knox KK. Subacute leukoencephalitis caused by CNS infection with human herpesvirus-6 manifesting as acute multiple sclerosis. *Neurology*. 1996;47:145-148.

59. Carter H, McKenna C, MacLeod R, Green R. Health professionals' responses to multiple sclerosis and motor neurone disease. *Palliat Med*. 1998;12:383-394.

60. Carter JL, Noseworthy JH. Ventilatory dysfunction in multiple sclerosis. *Clin Chest Med*. 1994;15:693-703.

61. Carton H, Vlietinck R, Debruyne J, et al. Risk of multiple sclerosis in relatives of patients in Flanders, Belgium. *J Neurol Neurosurg Psychiatry*. 1997;62:329-333.

62. Castano L, Eisenbarth GS. Type-1 diabetes: a chronic autoimmune disease of human, mouse, and rat. *Annu Rev Immunol*. 1990;8:647-679.

63. Chandrasoma P, Taylor CR. *Concise Pathology*. Stamford, Connecticut: Appleton & Lange; 1998.

64. Chataway J, Feakes R, Coraddu F, et al. The genetics of multiple sclerosis: principles, background and updated results of the United Kingdom systematic genome screen. *Brain*. 1998;121:1869-1887.

65. Chatterjee A, Yapundich R, Palmer CA, Marson DC, Mitchell GW. Leukoencephalopathy associated with cobalamin deficiency. *Neurology*. 1996;46:832-834.

66. Chaudhuri KR, Appiah-Kubi LS, Trenkwalder C. Restless legs syndrome. *J Neurol Neurosurg Psychiatry*. 2001;71:143-146.

67. Chew LD, Fihn SD. Bacterial infections of the urinary tract in women. In: Conn HF, ed. *Conn's Current Therapy*. Philadelphia, PA: W.B. Saunders;2000:662-666.

68. Coates T, Slavotinek JP, Rischmueller M, et al. Cerebral white matter lesions in primary Sjogren's syndrome: a controlled study. *J Rheumatol*. 1999;26:1301-1305.

69. Cohen JA. *MS and Its Masquerades: Diagnostic Dilemmas*. St. Paul, MN: American Academy of Neurology; 2000.

70. Coffeen CM, McKenna CE, Koeppen AH, et al. Genetic localization of an autosomal dominant leukodystrophy mimicking chronic progressive multiple sclerosis to chromosome 5q31. *Hum Mol Genet*. 2000;9:787-793.

71. Comi G, Filippi M, Barkhof F, et al. Effect of early interferon treatment on conversion to definite multiple sclerosis: a randomised study. *Lancet*. 2001;357:1576-1582.

72. Comi G, Filippi M, Wolinsky JS. European/Canadian multicenter, double-blind, randomized, placebo-controlled study of the effects of glatiramer acetate on magnetic resonance imaging—measured disease activity and burden in patients with relapsing multiple sclerosis. European/Canadian Glatiramer Acetate Study Group. *Ann Neurol*. 2001;49:290-297.

73. Compston A. Distribution of multiple sclerosis. In: Compston A, Ebers G, Lassman H, McDonald I, Matthews B, Wekerle H, eds. *McAlpine's Multiple Sclerosis*. London: Churchill Livingstone; 1998a:63-100.

74. Compston A. Genetic susceptibility to multiple sclerosis. In: Compston A, Ebers G, Lassman H, McDonald I, Matthews B, Wekerle, eds. *McAlpine's Multiple Sclerosis*. London: Churchill Livingstone; 1998b:101-142.

75. Compston A, Ebers G, Lassmann H, McDonald I, Matthews B, Wekerle H, eds. *McAlpine's Multiple Sclerosis*. London: Churchill Livingstone;1998c.

76. Confavreux C, Hutchinson M, Hours MM, et al. Rate of pregnancy-related relapse in multiple sclerosis. Pregnancy in Multiple Sclerosis Group. *N Engl J Med*. 1998;339:285-291.

77. Confavreux C. Combination therapies. In: Rudick RA, Goodkin DE, eds. *Multiple Sclerosis Therapeutics*. London: Blackwell Science Inc; 1999:395-413.

78. Confavreux C, Vukusic S, Moreau T, Adeleine P. Relapses and progression of disability in multiple sclerosis. *N Engl J Med*. 2000;343:1430-1438.

79. Confavreux C, Suissa S, Saddier P, Bourdes V, Vukusic S. Vaccinations and the risk of relapse in multiple sclerosis. Vaccines in Multiple Sclerosis Study Group. *N Engl J Med*. 2001;344:319-326.

80. Cook SD. *Handbook of Multiple Sclerosis (Neurological Disease and Therapy, Vol 53)*. New York, NY: Marcel Dekker; 2001.

81. Correale J, Arias M, Gilmore W. Steroid hormone regulation of cytokine secretion by proteolipid protein-specific CD4+ T cell clones isolated from multiple sclerosis patients and normal control subjects. *J Immunol*. 1998;161:3365-3374.

82. Cote DN, Molony TB, Waxman J, Parsa D. Cogan's syndrome manifesting as sudden bilateral deafness: diagnosis and mangement. *South Med J*. 1993;86:1056-1060.

83. Coyle PK. Diagnosis and classification of inflammatory demyelinating disorders. In: Burks JS, Johnson KP, eds. *Multiple Sclerosis: Diagnosis, Medical Management, and Rehabilitation*. New York, NY: Demos Medical Publishing; 2000:81-97.

84. Coyle PK. Women's issues. In: Burks JS, Johnson KP, eds. *Multiple Sclerosis: Diagnosis, Medical Management, and Rehabilitation*. New York, NY: Demos Medical Publishing; 2000:505-514.

85. Coyle P, Durelli L. *Clinical Considerations in the Management of MS with Interferons*. Ithaca Center for Postgraduate Medical Education. Ithaca NY;2001.

86. Crimlisk HL. The little imitator—porphyria: a neuropsychiatric disorder. *J Neurol Neurosurg Psychiatry*. 1997;62:319-328.

87. Cuadrado MJ, Khamashta MA, Ballesteros A, Godfrey T, Simon MJ, Hughes GR. Can neurologic manifestations of Hughes (antiphospholipid) syndrome be distinguished from multiple sclerosis? Analysis of 27 patients and review of the literature. *Medicine*. 2000;79:57-68.

88. Cutcliffe JR. How do nurses inspire and instil hope in terminally ill HIV patients? *J Adv Nurs*. 1995;22:888-895.

89. Davidson A, Diamond B. Autoimmune diseases. *N Engl J Med*. 2001;345:340-350.

90. De Angelis LM. Primary central nervous system lymphoma imitates multiple sclerosis. *J Neurooncol*. 1990;9:177-181.

91. De Benedittis G, Lorenzetti A, Sina C, Bernasconi V. Magnetic resonance imaging in migraine and tension-type headache. *Headache*. 1995;35:264-268.

92. Deen HG, Nelson KD, Gonzales GR. Spinal dural arteriovenous fistula causing progressive myelopathy: clinical and imaging considerations. *Mayo Clin Proc*. 1994;69:83-84.

93. De Gasperi R, Gama Sosa MA, Sartorato E, Battistini S, Raghavan S, Kolodny EH. Molecular basis of late-life globoid cell leukodystrophy. *Hum Mutat*. 1999;14:256-262.

10

94. De Keyser J, Zwanikken C, Boon M. Effects of influenza vaccination and influenza illness on exacerbations in multiple sclerosis. *J Neurol Sci.* 1998;159:51-53.

95. Demeter LM. JC, BK, and other polyomaviruses: progressive multifocal leukoencephalopathy. In: Mandell GL, Bennett JE, Dolin R, eds. *Principles and Practice of Infectious Diseases.* New York, NY: Churchill Livingstone; 2000:1645-1651.

96. De Pippo KL, Holas MA, Reding MJ. Validation of the 3-oz water swallow test for aspiration following stroke. *Arch Neurol.* 1992;49: 1259-1261.

97. Dichgans M, Mayer M, Uttner I, et al. The phenotypic spectrum of CADASIL: clinical findings in 102 cases. *Ann Neurol.* 1998;44:731-739.

98. Dierich M. Bladder dysfunction. In: Burks JS, Johnson KP, eds. *Multiple Sclerosis: Diagnosis, Medical Management, and Rehabilitation.* New York, NY: Demos Medical Publishing; 2000:433-451.

99. Di Mauro S, Bonilla E, De Vivo DC. Does the patient have a mitochondrial encephalomyopathy? *J Child Neurol.* 1999; 14(suppl 1):S23-S35.

100. Dotti MT, Caputo N, Signorini E, Federico A. Magnetic resonance imaging findings in Leber's hereditary optic neuropathy. *Eur Neurol.* 1992;32:17-19.

101. Duprez TP, Grandin CB, Bonnier C, et al. Whipple disease confined to the central nervous system in childhood. *Am J Neuroradiol.* 1996;17:1589-1591.

102. Ebers GC, Sadovnick AD, Risch NJ. A genetic basis for familial aggregation in multiple sclerosis. Canadian Collaborative Study Group. *Nature.* 1995;377:150-151.

103. Ebers GC, Sandovnick DA. Epidemiology. In: Paty DW, Ebers GC, eds. *Multiple Sclerosis.* Philadelphia, PA: FA Davis; 1998:5-28.

104. Ebers GC. Immunology. In: Paty DW, Ebers GC, eds. *Multiple Sclerosis.* Philadelphia, PA: FA Davis; 1998:403-426.

105. Ebers G. Natural history of multiple sclerosis. In: Compston A, Ebers G, Lassmann H, eds. *McAlpine's Multiple Sclerosis.* London: Harcourt Brace; 1998:191-221.

106. Ebers G, Paty DW. Natural history studies and applications to clinical trials. In: Paty DW, Ebers GC, eds. *Multiple Sclerosis.* Philadelphia, PA: FA Davis; 1998:193-228.

107. Ebers GC. Preventing multiple sclerosis? *Lancet.* 2001;357:1547.

108. Edan G, Miller D, Clanet M, et al. Therapeutic effect of mitoxantrone combined with methylprednisolone in multiple sclerosis: a randomised multicentre study of active disease using MRI and clinical criteria. *J Neurol Neurosurg Psychiatry.* 1997;62:112-118.

109. Edan G, LePage E, Taurin G, et al. Safety profile of mitoxantrone in a cohort of 293 multiple sclerosis patients. *Neurology.* 2001;56 (suppl):A149.

110. Eidelman BH. Autonomic disorders. In: Burks JS, Johnson KP, eds. *Multiple Sclerosis: Diagnosis, Medical Management, and Rehabilitation.* New York, NY: Demos Medical Publishing; 2000:471-483.

111. Engell T. A clinical patho-anatomical study of clinically silent multiple sclerosis. *Acta Neurol Scand.* 1989;79:428-430.

112. Ernst T, Chang L, Walot I, Huff K. Physiologic MRI of a tumefactive multiple sclerosis lesion. *Neurology.* 1998;51:1486-1488.

113. Estanislao LB, Pachner AR. Spirochetal infection of the nervous system. *Neurol Clin.* 1999;17:783-800.

114. Fazekas F, Strasser-Fuchs S, Gold R, Hartung HP. Intravenous immunoglobulin. In: Rudick RA, Goodkin DE, eds. *Multiple Sclerosis Therapeutics.* London: Blackwell Science Inc; 1999:309-322.

115. Feasby TE, Hahn AF, Koopman WJ, Lee DH. Central lesions in chronic inflammatory demyelinating polyneuropathy: an MRI study. *Neurology.* 1990;40:476-478.

116. Ferguson B, Matyszak MK, Esiri MM, Perry VH. Axonal damage in acute multiple sclerosis lesions. *Brain.* 1997;120: 393-399.

117. Fernandez RE, Rothberg M, Ferencz G, Wujack D. Lyme disease of the CNS: MR imaging findings in 14 cases. *Am J Neuroradiol.* 1990;11:479-481.

118. Filippi M, Paty DW, Kappos L, et al. Correlations between changes in disability and T2-weighted brain MRI activity in multiple sclerosis: a follow-up study. *Neurology.* 1995;45:255-260.

119. Filley CM, Kleinschmidt-De Masters BK. Toxic leukoencephalopathy. *N Engl J Med.* 2001;345:425-432.

120. Fink JK, Hedera P. Hereditary spastic paraplegia: genetic heterogeneity and genotype-phenotype correlation. *Sem Neurol.* 1999;19:301-309.

121. Fisher JS, Priore RL, Jacobs LD, et al. Neuropsychological effects of interferon beta-1a in relapsing multiple sclerosis. Multiple Sclerosis Collaborative Research Group. *Ann Neurol.* 2000;48:885-892.

122. Flachenecker P, Moriabadi N, Niewiesk S, Rieckmann P. Immunization and multiple sclerosis: clinical and immunological implications. *International Multiple Sclerosis Journal.* 2001;7:79-87.

123. Ford CC. Glatiramer acetate. In: Rudick RA, Goodkin DE, eds. *Multiple Sclerosis Therapeutics.* London: Blackwell Science Inc; 1999:277-297.

124. Freeman JA, Langdon DW, Hobart JC, Thompson AJ. Inpatient rehabilitation in multiple sclerosis: do the benefits carry over into the community? *Neurology.* 1999;52:50-56.

125. Frohman EM. Treatment for patients with relapsing-remitting multiple slcerosis. In: Rudick RA, Goodkin DE, eds. *Multiple Sclerosis Therapeutics.* London: Blackwell Science Inc; 1999:415-442.

126. Frohman EM, Zimmerman CF, Frohman TC. Neuro-ophthalmic signs and symptoms. In: Burks JS, Johnson KP, eds. *Multiple Sclerosis: Diagnosis, Medical Management, and Rehabilitation.* New York, NY: Demos Medical Publishing;2000:341-375.

127. Gahl WA. New therapies for Fabry's disease. *N Engl J Med.* 2001;345:55-57.

128. Gallucci M, Amicarelli I, Rossi A, et al. MR imaging of white matter lesions in uncomplicated alcoholism. *J Comput Assist Tomogr.* 1989;13:395-398.

129. Gardner P, Peter G. Recommended schedules for routine immunization of children and adults. *Infect Dis Clin North Am.* 2001;15:1-18.

130. Gass A, Filippi M, Grossman RI. The contribution of MRI in the differential diagnosis of posterior fossa damage. *J Neurol Sci.* 2000;(suppl 1):172:S43-S49.

131. Genis D, Matilla T, Volpini V, et al. Clinical, neuropathologic, and genetic studies of a large spinocerebellar ataxia type 1 (SCA 1) kindred: (CAG)n expansion and early premonitory signs and symptoms. *Neurology.* 1995;45:24-30.

10

132. Ghezzi A, Filippi M, Falini A, Zaffaroni M. Cerebral involvement in celiac disease: a serial MRI study in a patient with brainstem and cerebellar symptoms. *Neurology.* 1997;49:1447-1450.

133. Giang DW, Grow VM, Mooney C, et al. Clinical diagnosis of multiple sclerosis. The impact of magnetic resonance imaging and ancillary testing. Rochester-Toronto Magnetic Resonance Study Group. *Arch Neurol.* 1994;51:61-66.

134. Gilbert JJ, Sadler M. Unsuspected multiple sclerosis. *Arch Neurol.* 1983;40:533-536.

135. Goodkin DE, Jacobsen DW, Galvez N, Daughtry M, Secic M, Green R. Serum cobalamin deficiency is uncommon in multiple sclerosis. *Arch Neurol.* 1994;51:1110-1114.

136. Goodkin DE, Rudick RA, Vander Brug-Medendorp S, et al. Low-dose (7.5 mg) oral methotrexate reduces the rate of progression in chronic progressive multiple sclerosis. *Ann Neurol.* 1995;37:30-40.

137. Goodkin DE, Kinkel RP, Weinstock-Guttman B, et al. A phase II study of i.v. methylprednisolone in secondary-progressive multiple sclerosis. *Neurology.* 1999;52:896-897.

138. Gow PJ, Smallwood RA, Angus PW, Smith AL, Wall AJ, Sewell RB. Diagnosis of Wilson's disease: an experience over three decades. *Gut.* 2000;46:415-419.

139. Grand MG, Kaine J, Fulling K, et al. Cerebroretinal vasculopathy. A new hereditary syndrome. *Ophthalmology.* 1988;95:649-659.

140. Gray F, Chimelli L, Mohr M, Clavelou P, Scaravilli F, Poirier J. Fulminating multiple slcerosis-like leukoencephalopathy revealing human immunodeficiency virus infection. *Neurology.* 1991;41:105-109.

141. Green R, Kinsella LJ. Current concepts in the diagnosis of cobalamin deficiency. *Neurology.* 1995;45:1435-1440.

142. Green R, Miller JW. Folate deficiency beyond megaloblastic anemia: hyperhomocysteinemia and other manifestations of dysfunctional folate status. *Semin Hematol.* 1999;36:47-64.

143. Gregerson PK. Discordance for autoimmunity in monozygotic twins: Are "identical" twins really identical? *Arthritis and Rheumatism.* 1993;36:1185-1192.

144. Gross RE, Lozano AM. Advances in neurostimulation for movement disorders. *Neurol Res.* 2000;22:247-258.

145. Gunkle GM, Popper JG. *Incidental Heros: Disabling the Myths About Multiple Sclerosis.* New York, NY: National Multiple Sclerosis Society;1999.

146. Gutmann DH, Fischbeck KH, Sergott RC. Hereditary retinal vasculopathy with cerebral white matter lesions. *Am J Med Genet.* 1989;34:217-220.

147. Guyer DR, Gragoudas ES, Spaide RF, Starr CE. Central serous chorioretinopathy. In: Albert DM, Jakobiec FA, eds. *Principles and Practice of Opthalmology.* Philadelphia, PA: WB Saunders; 2000:1974-1982.

148. Guyer DR, Tretter T, D'Amico DJ, Ciardella AP. Lebers' idiopathic stellate neuroretinitis. In: Albert DM, Jakobiec FA, eds. *Principles and Practice of Ophthalmology.* Philadelphia, PA: WB Saunders; 2000:1965-1969.

149. Hadjimichael O, Vollmer TL. Adherence to injection therapy in multiple sclerosis: patient survey. *Neurology.* 2000;52(suppl 2):A549.

150. Hadjivassiliou M, Grunewald RA, Chattopadhyay AK, et al. Clinical, radiological, neurophysiological, and neuropathological characteristics of gluten ataxia. *Lancet*. 1998;352:1582-1585.

151. Hagenkotter B, Forster J, Ferbert A. Bickerstaff encephalitis. Clinical and magnetic resonance follow-up studies (German). *Nervenarzt*. 1998;69:892-895.

152. Hahn BH. Pathogenesis of systemic lupus erythematosus. In: Ruddy S, Harris ED, Sledge CB, eds. *Kelley's Textbook of Rheumatology* (2-Volume Set). New York, NY: WB Saunders Co; 2001:1089-1103.

153. Harding AE, Sweeney MG, Miller DH, et al. Occurrence of a multiple sclerosis-like illness in women who have a Leber's hereditary optic neuropathy mitochondrial DNA mutation. *Brain*. 1992;115:979-989.

154. Harris DE, Enterline DS, Tien RD. Neurosyphilis in patients with AIDS. *Neuroimaging Clin N Am*. 1997;7:215-221.

155. Harris EC, Barraclough BM. Suicide as an outcome for medical disorders. *Medicine*. 1994;73:281-296.

156. Hartung HP, Gonsette R, Morrissey S, Krapf H, Fazekas F. Mitoxantrone. In: Rudick RA, Goodkin DE, eds. *Multiple Sclerosis Therapeutics*. London: Blackwell Science Inc; 1999:335-348.

157. Hawkins CP, Wolinsky JS, eds. *Principles of Treatments in Multiple Sclerosis*. Oxford: Butterworth-Heinemann; 2000.

158. Heesen C, Bergmann M, Figge C, Loschke S, Feldmann M. Intravascular lymphomatosis of the nervous system—case report and review of the literature (German). *Fortschr Neurol Psychiatr*. 1996;64:234-241.

159. Herndon RM, Rudick RA. Multiple sclerosis. The spectrum of severity. *Arch Neurol*. 1983;40:531-532.

160. Herndon RM. Pathology and Pathophysiology. In: Burks JS, Johnson KP, eds. *Multiple Sclerosis: Diagnosis, Medical Management, and Rehabilitation*. New York, NY: Demos Medical Publishing; 2000:35-45.

161. Higgins JJ, Loveless JM, Goswami S, et al. An atypical intronic deletion widens the spectrum of mutations in hereditary spastic paraplegia. *Neurology*. 2001;56:1482-1485.

162. Holland NJ. Bowel management. In: van den Noort S, Holland NJ, eds. *Multiple Sclerosis in Clinical Practice*. New York, NY: Demos Medical Publishing; 1999:81-88.

163. Horvath R, Abicht A, Shoubridge EA, et al. Leber's hereditary optic neuropathy presenting as multiple sclerosis-like disease of the CNS. *J Neurol*. 2000;247:65-67.

164. Houtman JJ, Fleming JO. Pathogenesis of mouse hepatitis virus-induced demyelination. *J Neurovirol*. 1996;2:361-376.

165. Howell JB. Behavioural breathlessness. *Thorax*. 1990;45:287-292.

166. Huang CC, Wai YY, Chu NS, et al. Mitochondrial encephalomyopathies: CT and MRI findings and correlations with clinical features. *Eur Neurol*. 1995;35:199-205.

167. Hurley RA, Tomimoto H, Akiguchi I, Fisher RE, Taber KH. Binswanger's disease: an ongoing controversy. *J Neuropsychiatry Clin Neurosci*. 2000;12:301-304.

168. Hussain I, Fowler C. The cause and management of bladder, sexual and bowel symptoms. In: Hawkins C, Wolinsky JS, eds. *Principles of Treatments in Multiple Sclerosis*. Oxford: Butterworth-Heinemann Medical; 2000:258-281.

10

169. Hynson JL, Kornberg AJ, Coleman LT, Shield L, Harvey AS, Kean MJ. Clinical and neuroradiologic features of acute disseminated encephalomyelitis in children. *Neurology*. 2001;56:1308-1312.

170. Inuzuka T. Autoantibodies in paraneoplastic neurological syndrome. *Am J Med Sci*. 2000;319:217-226.

171. Jacobs LD, Beck RW, Simon JH, et al. Intramuscular interferon beta-1a therapy initiated during a first demyelinating event in multiple sclerosis. CHAMPS Study Group. *N Engl J Med*. 2000;343:898-904.

172. Jacobsen M, Schweer D, Ziegler A, et al. A point mutation in PTPRC is associated with the development of multiple sclerosis. *Nat Genet*. 2000;26:495-499.

173. Jaster JH, Bertorini TE, Dohan FC, et al. Solitary focal demyelination in the brain as a paraneoplastic disorder. *Med Pediatr Oncol*. 1996;26:111-115.

174. Jeffery DR, Mandler RN, Davis LE. Transverse myelitis. Retrospective analysis of 33 cases, with differentiation of cases associated with multiple sclerosis and parainfectious events. *Arch Neurol*. 1993;50:532-535.

175. Jeffery DR. Pain and dysesthesia. In Burks JS, Johnson KP, eds. *Multiple Sclerosis: Diagnosis, Medical Management, and Rehabilitation*. New York, NY: Demos Medical Publishing; 2000:425-431.

176. Jen J, Cohen AH, Yue Q, et al. Hereditary endotheliopathy with retinopathy, nephropathy, and stroke (HERNS). *Neurology*. 1997;49:1322-1330.

177. Johnson KP, Brooks BR, Cohen JA. Copolymer 1 reduces relapse rate and improves disability in relapsing-remitting multiple sclerosis: results of a phase III multicenter, double-blind placebo-controlled trial. The Copolymer 1 Multiple Sclerosis Study Group. *Neurology*. 1995;45:1268-1276.

178. Johnson KP. Therapy of relapsing forms. In: Burks JS, Johnson KP, eds. *Multiple Sclerosis: Diagnosis, Medical Management, and Rehabilitation*. New York, NY: Demos Medical Publishing; 2000:167-175.

179. Joy JE, Johnston RB, eds. *Multiple Sclerosis: Current Status and Strategies for the Future*. Washington, DC: National Academy Press; 2001.

180. Kalman B, Lublin FD, Alder H. Mitochondrial DNA mutations in multiple sclerosis. *Mult Scler*. 1995;1:32-36.

181. Kanner R. Treatment of chronic pain. In: Rudick RA, Goodkin DE, eds. *Multiple Sclerosis Therapeutics*. London: Blackwell Science Inc; 1999:541-546.

182. Karussis D, Leker RR, Ashkenazi A, Abramsky O. A subgroup of multiple sclerosis patients with anticardiolipin antibodies and unusual clinical manifestations: do they represent a new nosological entity? *Ann Neurol*. 1998;44:629-634.

183. Kastrukoff LF, Rice GPA. Virology. In: Paty DW, Ebers GC, eds. *Multiple Sclerosis*. Philadelphia, PA: FA Davis;1998:370-402.

184. Katz JD, Ropper AH. Progressive necrotic myelopathy: clinical course in 9 patients. *Arch Neurol*. 2000;57:355-361.

185. Keime-Guibert F, Napolitano M, Delattre JY. Neurological complications of radiotherapy and chemotherapy. *J Neurol*. 1998;245:695-708.

186. Kelly R. Clinical aspects of multiple sclerosis. In: Vinken PJ, Bruyn GW, Klawans HL, Koetsier JC, eds. *Handbook of Clinical Neurology: Volume 47, Demyelinating Diseases.* Amsterdam: Elsevier, 1985:49-78.

187. Kerslake R, Rowe D, Worthington BS. CT and MR imaging of CNS lymphomatoid granulomatosis. *Neuroradiology.* 1991;33:269-271.

188. Kesselring J, Omerod IEC, Miller DH, du Boulay GHEP, McDonald WI. *Magnetic Resonance Imaging in Multiple Sclerosis.* New York, NY: Theime Medical Publishers;1989.

189. Kesselring J, Miller DH, Robb SA, et al. Acute disseminated encephalomyelitis. MRI findings and the distinction from multiple sclerosis. *Brain.* 1990;113:291-302.

190. Khan OA, Bauserman SC, Rothman MI, Aldrich EF, Panitch HS. Concurrence of multiple sclerosis and brain tumor: clinical considerations. *Neurology.* 1997;48:1330-1333.

191. Khan OA, Tselis AC, Kamholz JA, Garbern JY, Lewis RA, Lisak RP. A prospective, open-label treatment trial to compare the effect of IFN beta-1a (Avonex), IFNbeta-1b (Betaseron), and glatiramer acetate (Copaxone) on the relapse rate in relapsing-remitting multiple sclerosis. *Eur J Neurol.* 2001;8:141-148.

192. Kidd D, Steuer A, Denman AM, Rudge P. Neurological complications in Behcet's syndrome. *Brain.* 1999;122:2183-2194.

193. Kim S, Liva SM, Dalal MA, Verity MA, Voskuhl RR. Estriol ameliorates autoimmune demyelinating disease: implications for multiple sclerosis. *Neurology.* 1999;52:1230-1238.

194. King PH, Bragdon AC. MRI reveals multiple reversible cerebral lesions in an attack of acute intermittent porphyria. *Neurology.* 1991;41:1300-1302.

195. Kinkel RP. Methylprednisolone. In: Rudick RA, Goodkin DE, eds. *Multiple Sclerosis Therapeutics.* London: Blackwell Science Inc; 1999:349-370.

196. Kita M. Treatment of spasticity. In: Rudick RA, Goodkin DE, eds. *Multiple Sclerosis Therapeutics.* London: Blackwell Science Inc; 1999:475-488.

197. Klockgether T, Skalej M, Wedekind D, et al. Autosomal dominant cerebellar ataxia type 1. MRI-based volumetry of posterior fossa structures and basal ganglia in spinocerebellar ataxia types 1, 2 and 3. *Brain.* 1998;121:1687-1693.

198. Koizumi J, Ofuku K, Sakuma K, Shiraishi H, Iio M, Nawano S. CNS changes in Usher's syndrome with mental disorder: CT, MRI and PET findings. *J Neurol Neurosurg Psychiatry.* 1988;51:987-990.

199. Korte JH, Bom EP, Vos LD, Breuer TJ, Wondergem JH. Balo concentric sclerosis: MR diagnosis. *Am J Neuroradiol.* 1994;15:1284-1285.

200. Kotzin BL. Autoimmunity. In: Ruddy S, Harris ED, Sledge CB, eds. *Kelley's Textbook of Rheumatology* (2-Volume Set). New York, NY: WB Saunders Co; 2001:305-319.

201. Kovalchik MT. "Playing God" as an act of hope. *Ann Intern Med.* 1992;117:1060.

202. Kraushar MF, Miller EM. Central serous choroidopathy misdiagnosed as a manifestation of multiple sclerosis. *Ann Ophthalmol.* 1982;14:215-218.

10

203. Krupp LB, Elkins LE. Fatigue. In: Burks JS, Johnson KP, eds. *Multiple Sclerosis: Diagnosis, Medical Management, and Rehabilitation.* New York, NY: Demos Medical Publishing; 2000:291-297.

204. Kumar SR, Mone AP, Gray LC, Troost BT. Central pontine myelinolysis: delayed changes on neuroimaging. *J Neuroimaging.* 2000;10:169-172.

205. Kuroda Y, Matsui M, Yukitake M, et al. Assessment of MRI criteria for MS in Japanese MS and HAM/TSP. *Neurology.* 1995;45:30-33.

206. Kurtzke JF. Geography in multiple sclerosis. *J Neurol.* 1977; 215:1-26.

207. Kurtzke JF, Beebe GW, Nagler B, Kurland LT, Auth TL: Studies on the natural history of multiple sclerosis. VIII. Early prognostic features of the later course of the illness. *J Chron Diseases.* 1977;30:819-830.

208. LaRocca NG. Cognitive and emotional disorders. In: Burks JS, Johsnon KP, eds. *Multiple Sclerosis: Diagnosis, Medcial Management, and Rehabilitation.* New York, NY: Demos Medical Publishing; 2000:405-423.

209. Lassmann H, Wekerle H. Experimental models of multiple sclerosis. In: Compston A, Ebers G, Lassmann H eds. *McAlpine's Multiple Sclerosis.* London, Harcourt Brace; 1998:409-433.

210. Lee SH, Yoon PH, Park SJ, Kim DI. MRI findings in neuro-behcet's disease. *Clin Radiol.* 2001;56:485-494.

211. Lie JT. Malignant angioendotheliomatosis (intravascular lymphomatosis) clinically simulating primary angiitis of the central nervous system. *Arthritis Rheum.* 1992;35:831-834.

212. Litwiller SE. Treatment of bladder and sexual dysfunction. In: Rudick RA, Goodkin DE, eds. *Multiple Sclerosis Therapeutics.* London: Blackwell Science Inc; 1999:489-516.

213. Lossos A, Barash V, Soffer D, et al. Hereditary branching enzyme dysfunction in adult polyglucosan body disease: a possible metabolic cause in two patients. *Ann Neurol.* 1991;30:655-662.

214. Lublin FD, Reingold SC. Defining the clinical course of multiple sclerosis: results of an international survey. National Multiple Sclerosis Society (USA) Advisory Committee on Clinical Trials of New Agents in Multiple Sclerosis. *Neurology.* 1996;46:907-911.

215. Lucchinetti C, Bruck W, Parisi J, Scheithauer B, Rodriguez M, Lassmann H. Heterogeneity of multiple sclerosis lesions: implications for the pathogenesis of demyelination. *Ann Neurol.* 2000;47:707-717.

216. Lucchinetti CF, Kimmel DW, Pavelko K, Rodriguez M. 5-Fluorouracil and levamisole exacerbate demyelination in susceptible mice infected with Theiler's virus. *Exp Neurol.* 1997;147:123-129.

217. Lucchinetti C. The spectrum of idiopathic inflammatory demyelinating disease. In: Weinshenker B. *Acute Leukoencephalopathies.* St. Paul, MN: American Academy of Neurology; 2000:14-25.

218. Ludwin SK. Understanding multiple sclerosis: lessons from pathology. *Ann Neurol.* 2000;47:691-693.

219. Lynch SG, Digrek, Rose JW. Usher's syndrome with a multiple sclerosis-like illness. *J Neuro-Ophthal.* 1994;14:34-37.

220. Lynn J, Rammohan KW, Bornstein RA, Kissel JT. Central nervous system involvement in the eosinophilia-myalgia syndrome. *Arch Neurol.* 1992;49:1082-1085.

221. Mackenzie IR, Carrigan DR, Wiley CA. Chronic myelopathy associated with human herpesvirus-6. *Neurology*. 1995;45:2015-2017.

222. Maloni H, Schapiro RT. Pain. In: van den Noort S, Holland NJ. *Multiple Sclerosis in Clinical Practice*. New York, NY: Demos Medical Publishing; 1999:57-66.

223. Mandler RN, Ahmed W, Dencoff JE. Devic's neuromyelitis optica: a prospective study of seven patients treated with prednisone and azathioprine. *Neurology*. 1998;51:1219-1220.

224. Manzel K, Tranel D, Cooper G. Cognitive and behavioral abnormalities in a case of central nervous system Whipple disease. *Arch Neurol*. 2000;57:399-403.

225. Markus H. Personal communication, 2001.

226. Martino G, Furlan R, Brambilla E, et al. Cytokines and immunity in multiple sclerosis: the dual signal hypothesis. *J Neuroimmunol*. 2000;109:3-9.

227. Masdeu JC, Moreira J, Trasi S, Visintainer P, Cavaliere R, Grundman M. The open ring. A new imaging sign in demyelinating disease. *J Neuroimaging*. 1996;6:104-107.

228. Matthews B. Differential diagnosis of multiple sclerosis and related disorders. In: Compston A, Ebers G, Lassmann H, eds. *McAlpine's Multiple Sclerosis*. London: Harcourt Brace; 1998:223-250.

229. Matthews B. Symptoms and signs of multiple sclerosis. In: Compston A, Ebers G, Lassmann H, eds. *McAlpine's Multiple Sclerosis*. London: Harcourt Brace; 1998:145-190.

230. Mattingly G, Baker K, Zorumski CF, Figiel GS. Multiple sclerosis and ECT: possible value of gadolinium-enhanced magnetic resonance scans for identifying high-risk patients. *J Neuropsychiatry Clin Neruosci*. 1992;4:145-151.

231. McAlpine D, Lumsden CE, Acheson ED. *Multiple Sclerosis*. Edinburgh: Churchill Limestone;1972.

232. McDermott C, White K, Bushby K, Shaw P. Hereditary spastic paraparesis: a review of new developments. *J Neurol Neurosurg Psychiatry*. 2000;69:150-160.

233. McDonald WI. Diagnostic methods and investigations in multiple sclerosis. In: Compston A, Ebers G, Lassmann H, eds. *McAlpine's Multiple Sclerosis*. London: Harcourt Brace; 1998:251-279.

234. McDonald WI, Compston A, Edan G, et al. Recommended diagnostic criteria for multiple sclerosis: guidelines from the International Panel on the diagnosis of multiple sclerosis. *Ann Neurol*. 2001;50:121-127.

235. Meadows J, Kraut M, Guarnieri M, Haroun RL, Carson BS. Asymptomatic Chiari Type 1 malformations identified on magnetic resonance imaging. *J Neurosurg*. 2000;92:920-926.

236. Merino JG, Hachinski V. Leukoaraiosis: reifying rarefaction. *Arch Neurol*. 2000;57:925-926.

237. Millefiorini E, Gasperini C, Pozzilli C, et al. Randomized placebo-controlled trial of mitoxantrone in relapsing-remitting multiple sclerosis: 24-month clinical and MRI outcome. *J Neurol*. 1997;224:153-159.

238. Miller A, Bourdette D, Cohen JA, et al. Multiple sclerosis. *Continuum*. 1999;5:41-42.

239. Miller A. Paroxysmal disorders. In: Burks JS, Johnson KP, eds. *Multiple Sclerosis: Diagnosis, Medical Management, and Rehabilitation*. New York, NY: Demos Medical Publishing; 2000:377-384.

10

240. Mills RW, Schoolfield L. Acute transverse myelitis associated with *Mycoplasma pneumoniae* infection: a case report and review of the literature. *Pediatr Infect Dis J.* 1992;11:228-231.

241. Milo R, Panitch H. Glatiramer acetate or interferon-beta for multiple sclerosis? A guide to drug choice. *CNS Drugs.* 1999;11:289-306.

242. Montgomery EB, Baker KB, Kinkel RP, Barnett G. Chronic thalamic stimulation for the tremor of multiple sclerosis. *Neurology.* 1999;53:625-628.

243. Morel L, Croker BP, Blenman KR, et al. Genetic reconstitution of systemic lupus erythematosus immunopathology with polycongenic murine strains. *Proc Natl Acad Sci.* 2000;97:6670-6675.

244. Morrison J. Managing somatization disorder. *Dis Mon.* 1990;36:537-591.

245. Morrissey SP, Miller DH, Kendall BE, et al. The significance of brain magnetic resonance imaging abnormalities at presentation with clinically isolated syndromes suggestive of multiple sclerosis. A 5-year follow-up study. *Brain.* 1993;116:135-146.

246. Morrissey SP, Miller DH, Hermaszewski R, et al. Magnetic resonance imaging of the central nervous system in Behcet's disease. *Eur Neurol.* 1993;33:287-293.

247. Moser HW. *Diagnosis and Therapy of Leukodystrophies.* American Academy of Neurology; 2000.

248. Munoz A, Mateos F, Simon R, Garcia-Silva MT, Cabello S, Arenas J. Mitochondrial diseases in children: neuroradiological and clinical features in 17 patients. *Neuroradiology.* 1999;41:920-928.

249. Murray JT. The history of multiple sclerosis. In: Burks JS, Johnson KP, eds. *Multiple Sclerosis: Diagnosis, Medical Management, and Rehabilitation.* New York, NY: Demos Medical Publishing; 2000:1-32.

250. Mushlin AI, Detsky AS, Phelps CE, et al. The accuracy of magnetic resonance imaging in patients with suspected multiple sclerosis. The Rochester-Toronto Magnetic Resonance Imaging Study Group. *JAMA.* 1993;269:3146-3151.

251. Nadeau SE. Diagnostic approach to central and peripheral nervous system vasculitis. *Neurol Clin.* 1997;15:759-777.

252. Nassar NN, Smith JW. Bacterial infections of the urinary tract in men. In: Conn HF, ed. *Conn's Current Therapy.* Philadelphia, PA: W.B. Saunders; 2000:661-662.

253. National Multiple Sclerosis Society. *Multiple Sclerosis in 2000: A Model of Psychosocial Support.* New York, NY:2000.

254. National Multiple Sclerosis Society. Research Update, August 3, 2001.

255. Natowicz MR, Bejjani B. Genetic disorders that masquerade as multiple sclerosis. *Am J Med Genetics.* 1994;49:149-169.

256. Natowicz MR, Prence EM, Chaturvedi P, Newburg DS. Urine sulfatides and the diagnosis of metachromatic leukodystrophy. *Clin Chem.* 1996;42:232-238.

257. Naviaux RK. Mitochondrial DNA disorders. *Eur J Pediatr.* 2000;159(suppl 3):S219-S226.

258. Nielsen JE, Krabbe K, Jennum P, et al. Autosomal dominant pure spastic paraplegia: a clinical, paraclinical, and genetic study. *J Neurol Neurosurg Psychiatry.* 1998;64:61-66.

259. Nies AS. Principles of therapeutics. In: Hardman JG, Limbird LE, eds. *Goodman & Gilman's The Pharmacological Basis of Therapeutics.* New York, NY: McGraw-Hill Professional Publishing; 2001:45-66.

260. Niranjan A, Kondziolka D, Baser S, Heyman R, Lunsford LD. Functional outcomes after gamma knife thalamotomy for essential tremor and MS-related tremor. *Neurology.* 2000;55:443-446.

261. Noseworthy JH. Progress in determining the causes and treatment of multiple sclerosis. *Nature.* 1999;(suppl)399:A40-A47.

262. Noseworthy JH, Lucchinetti C, Rodriguez M, Weinshenker BG. Multiple sclerosis. *N Engl J Med.* 2000;343:938-952.

263. O'Riordan JI, Thompson AJ, Kingsley DP, et al. The prognostic value of brain MRI in clinically isolated syndromes of the CNS. A 10-year follow-up. *Brain.* 1998;121:495-503.

264. O'Sullivan M, Jarosz JM, Martin RJ, Deasy N, Powell JF, Markus HS. MRI hyperintensities of the temporal lobe and external capsule in patients with CADASIL. *Neurology.* 2001;56:628-634.

265. Obach V, Gonzalez-Menacho J, Vidal S, Lomena F, Graus F. Tl-201 SPECT in pseudotumoral multiple sclerosis. *Clin Nucl Med.* 1999;24:186-188.

266. Oksenberg JR, Baranzini SE, Barcellos LF, Hauser SL. Multiple sclerosis: genomic rewards. *J Neuroimmunol.* 2001; 113:171-184.

267. Okumura A, Hayakawa F, Kato T, Kuno K, Watanabe K. MRI findings in patients with spastic cerebral palsy. I: Correlation with gestational age at birth. *Dev Med Child Neurol.* 1997;39:363-368.

268. Ophoff RA, DeYoung J, Service SK, et al. Hereditary vascular retinopathy, cerebroretinal vasculopathy, and hereditary endotheliopathy with retinopathy, nephropathy, and stroke map to a single locus on chromosome 3p21.1-p21.3. *Am J Hum Genet.* 2001;69:447-453.

269. Oppenheim C, Galanaud D, Samson Y, et al. Can diffusion weighted magnetic resonance imaging help differentiate stroke from stroke-like events in MELAS? *J Neurol Neurosurg Psychiatry.* 2000;69:248-250.

270. Optic Neuritis Study Group. The 5-year risk of MS after optic neuritis. Experience of the optic neuritis treatment trial. *Neurology.* 1997;49:1404-1413.

271. Ormerod IE, Harding AE, Miller DH, et al. Magnetic resonance imaging in degenerative ataxic disorders. *J Neurol Neurosurg Psychiatry.* 1994;57:51-57.

272. Owens GP, Kraus H, Burgoon MP, Smith-Jensen T, Devlin ME, Gilden DH. Restricted use of VH4 germline segments in an acute multiple sclerosis brain. *Ann Neurol.* 1998;43:236-243.

273. Owens T, Wekerle H, Antel J. Genetic models for CNS inflammation. *Nat Med.* 2001;7:161-166.

274. Panitch HS. Influence of infection on exacerbations of multiple sclerosis. *Ann Neurol.* 1994;36(suppl):S25-S28.

275. Panitch HS, Hirsch RL, Schindler J, Johnson KP. Treatment of multiple sclerosis with gamma interferon: exacerbations associated with activation of the immune system. *Neurology.* 1987;37:1097-1102.

276. Papo T, Biousse V, Lehoang P, et al. Susac syndrome. *Medicine.* 1998;77:3-11.

277. Paszner B, Petkau J, Oger J. Impact of antibodies to interferon-beta during treatment of multiple sclerosis. In: Wagstaff A, ed. *Drug Treatment of Mutliple Sclerosis.* Auckland, NZ: Lippincott Williams & Wilkins Publishers; 2000:89-108.

278. Paty DW, Noseworthy JH, Ebers GC. Diagnosis of multiple sclerosis. In: Paty DW, Ebers GC, eds. *Multiple Sclerosis.* Philadelphia, PA: FA Davis;1998:48-134.

10

279. Paty DW, Moore GRW. Magnetic resonance imaging changes as living pathology in multiple sclerosis. In: Paty DW, Ebers GC, eds. *Multiple Sclerosis*. Philadelphia, PA: FA Davis;1998:328-369.

280. Paty DW, Ebers GC, eds. *Multiple Sclerosis*: Philadelphia, PA: FA Davis,1998c.

281. Paulson GW. Pseudo-multiple sclerosis. *South Med J.* 1996;89:301-304.

282. Paydarfar D, de la Monte SM. Case records of the Massachusetts General Hospital. Weekly clinicopathological exercises. Case 12-1997. A 50-year-old woman with multiple sclerosis and an enlarging frontal-lobe mass. *N Engl J Med.* 1997;336:1163-1171.

283. Pellecchia MT, Scala R, Filla A, De Michele G, Ciacci C, Barone P. Idiopathic cerebellar ataxia associated with celiac disease: lack of distinctive neurological features. *J Neurol Neurosurg Psychiatry.* 1999;66:32-35.

284. Percy AK, Nobrega FT, Kurland LT. Optic neuritis and multiple sclerosis. An epidemiologic study. *Arch Opthalmol.* 1972;87:135-139.

285. Perkins L, Perkins S. *Multiple Sclerosis: Your Legal Rights.* New York, NY: Demos Medical Publishing;1999.

286. Petajan JH, Gappmaier E, White AT, Spencer MK, Mino L, Hicks RW. Impact of aerobic training on fitness and quality of life in multiple sclerosis. *Ann Neurol.* 1996;39:432-441.

287. Peterson K, Rosenblum MK, Powers JM, Alvord E, Walker RW, Posner JB. Effect of brain irradiation on demyelinating lesions. *Neurology.* 1993;43:2105-2112.

288. Petty GW, Engel AG, Younge BR, et al. Retinocochleocerebral vasculopathy. *Medicine.* 1998;77:12-40.

289. Pfefferbaum A, Sullivan EV, Mathalon DH, Shear PK, Rosenbloom MJ, Lim KO. Longitudinal changes in magnetic resonance imaging brain volumes in abstinent and relapsed alcoholics. *Alcohol Clin Exp Res.* 1995;19:1177-1191.

290. Phillips JT. Genetics susceptibility models in multiple sclerosis. In: Rosenberg RN, Barchi RL, Dimauro S, Kunkel LM. *The Molecular and Genetic Basis of Neurological Disease.* Boston, MA: Butterworth-Heinemann; 1993:41-46.

291. *Physicians' Desk Reference.* Montvale, NJ: Medical Economics;2002.

292. Pickuth D, Spielmann RP, Heywang-Kobrunner SH. Role of radiology in the diagnosis of neurosarcoidosis. *Eur Radiol.* 2000;10:941-944.

293. Polman CH, Herndon RM, Pozzilli C. Interferons. In: Rudick RA, Goodkin DE, eds. *Multiple Sclerosis Therapeutics.* London: Blackwell Science Inc; 1999:243-276.

294. Polman CH, Uitdehaag BM. Drug treatment of multiple sclerosis. *BMJ.* 2000;321:490-494.

295. Polman CH, Thompson AJ, Murray TJ, McDonald WI. *Multiple Sclerosis: The Guide to Treatment and Management.* New York, NY: Demos Medical Publishing;2001.

296. Poser CM. The dissemination of multiple sclerosis: a Viking saga? A historical essay. *Ann Neurol.* 1994;36(suppl 2):S231-S243.

297. Poser CM. Misdiagnosis of multiple sclerosis and beta-interferon. *Lancet.* 1997;349:1916.

298. Poser CM. Interferon beta-1a during a first demyelinating event. *N Engl J Med.* 2001;344:229-230.

299. Post MJ, Yiannoutsos C, Simpson D, et al. Progressive multifocal leukoencephalopathy in AIDS: are there any MR findings useful to patient management and predictive of patient survival? AIDS Clinical Trials Group, 243 Team. *Am J Neuroradiol.* 1999;20:1896-1906.

300. Preskorn SH. *Outpatient Management of Depression: A Guide for the Primary-Care Practitioner.* Caddo, OK: Professional Communications Inc;1999.

301. Preul MC, Caramanos Z, Collins DL, et al. Accurate, noninvasive diagnosis of human brain tumors by using proton magnetic resonance spectroscopy. *Nat Med.* 1996;2:323-325.

302. Prineas JW, Connell F. The fine structure of chronically active multiple sclerosis plaques. *Neurology.* 1978;28(9 Pt 2):68-75.

303. PRISMS Study Group. Randomised double-blind placebo-controlled study of interferon beta-1a in relapsing/remitting multiple sclerosis. *Lancet.* 1998;352:1498-1504.

304. PRIMSMS-4: Long-term efficacy of interferon-beta-1a in relapsing MS. *Neurology.* 2001;56:1628-1636.

305. Prusiner SB. Shattuck lecture—neurodegenerative diseases and prions. *N Engl J Med.* 2001;344:1516-1526.

306. Purvin VA. Optic neuropathies for the neurologist. *Semin Neurol.* 2000;20:97-110.

307. Rafto SE, Milton WJ, Galetta SL, Grossman RI. Biopsy-confirmed CNS Lyme disease. MR appearance at 1.5 T. *Am J Neuroradiol.* 1990;11:482-484.

308. Rao SM. Neuropsychology of multiple sclerosis. *Curr Opin Neurol.* 1995;8:216-220.

309. Ridley A, Schapira K. Influence of surgical procedures on the course of multiple sclerosis. *Neurology.* 1961;11:81-92.

310. Ristori G, Buzzi MG, Sabatini U, et al. Use of Bacille Calmette-Guerin (BCG) in multiple sclerosis. *Neurology.* 1999;53:1588-1589.

311. Rivaud-Pechoux S, Durr A, Gaymard B, et al. Eye movement abnormalities correlate with genotype in autosomal dominant cerebellar ataxia type 1. *Ann Neurol.* 1998;43:297-302.

312. Rizzo JF, Lessell S. Risk of developing multiple sclerosis after uncomplicated optic neuritis: a long-term prospective study. *Neurology.* 1988;38:185-190.

313. Robertson NP, O'Riordan JI, Chataway J, et al. Offspring recurrence rates and clinical characteristics of conjugal multiple sclerosis. *Lancet.* 1997;349:1587-1590.

314. Rocca MA, Colombo B, Pratesi A, Comi G, Filippi M. A magnetization transfer imaging study of the brain in patients with migraine. *Neurology.* 2000;54:507-509.

315. Rodier G, Derouiche F, Bronner P, Cohen E. Eales disease with neurologic manifestation: differential diagnosis of multiple sclerosis. Report of two cases. *Presse Med.* 1999;28:1692-1694.

316. Roos RP. Controlling new prion diseases. *N Engl J Med.* 2001;344: 1548-1551.

317. Rorie KD, Stump DA, Jeffery DR. Effect of donepezil on cognitive function in patients with multiple sclerosis. *Neurology.* 2001;56 (suppl):A99.

318. Rosenbaum RB, Campbell SM, Rosenbaum JT. *Clinical Neurology of Rheumatic Diseases.* Boston, Mass: Butterworth-Heinemann, 1996.

10

319. Rudge P, Ali A, Cruickshank JK. Multiple sclerosis, tropical spastic paraparesis and HTLV-1 infection in Afro-Caribbean patients in the United Kingdom. *J Neurol Neurosurg Psychiatry*. 1991;54:689-694.

320. Rudick RA, Schiffer RB, Schwetz KM, Herndon RM. Multiple sclerosis. The problem of incorrect diagnosis. *Arch Neurol*. 1986;43:578-583.

321. Rudick RA, Fisher E, Lee JC, Simon J, Jacobs L. Use of the brain parenchymal fraction to measure whole brain atrophy in relapsing-remitting MS. Multiple Sclerosis Collaborative Research Group. *Neurology*. 1999;53:1698-1704.

322. Rudick RA. Disease-modifying drugs for relapsing-remitting multiple sclerosis and future directions for multiple sclerosis therapeutics. *Arch Neurol*. 1999;56:1079-1084.

323. Rudick RA, Goodkin DE, eds. *Multiple Sclerosis Therapeutics*. London: Martin Dunitz;1999.

324. Rust RS. Multiple sclerosis, acute disseminated encephalomyelitis, and related conditions. *Semin Pediatr Neurol*. 2000;7:66-90.

325. Sadovnick AD, Ebers GC, Dyment DA, Risch NJ. Evidence for genetic basis of multiple sclerosis. The Canadian Collaborative Study Group. *Lancet*. 1996;347:1728-1730.

326. Sadovnick AD, Ebers GC. Epidemiology of multiple sclerosis: a critical overview. *Can J Neurol Sci*. 1993;20:17-29.

327. Sampson SM. Treating depression with selective serotonin reuptake inhibitors: a practical approach. *Mayo Clin Proc*. 2001;76:739-744.

328. Sastre-Garriga J, Reverter JC, Font J, Tintore M, Espinosa G, Montalban X. Anticardiolipin antibodies are not a useful screening tool in a nonselected large group of patients with multiple sclerosis. *Ann Neurol*. 2001;49:408-411.

329. Satoh JI, Tokumoto H, Kurohara K, Yukitake M, Matsui M, Kuroda Y. Adult-onset Krabbe disease with homozygous T1853C mutation in the galactocerebrosidase gene. Unusual MRI findings of corticospinal tract demyelination. *Neurology*. 1997;49:1392-1399.

330. Satya-Murti S, Howard L, Krohel G, Wolf B. The spectrum of neurologic disorder from vitamin E deficiency. *Neurology*. 1986;36:917-921.

331. Saunders AS, Aisen ML. Sexual dysfunction. In: Burks JS, Johnson KP, eds. *Multiple Sclerosis: Diagnosis, Medical Management, and Rehabilitation*. New York, NY: Demos Medcial Publishing; 2000:461-470.

332. Savarese DM, Gordon J, Smith TW, et al. Cerebral demyelination syndrome in a patient treated with 5-fluorouracil and levamisole. The use of thallium SPECT imaging to assist in noninvasive diagnosis—a case report. *Cancer*. 1996;77:387-394.

333. Schanke AK, Sundet K. Comprehensive driving assessment: neuropsychological testing and on-road evaluation of brain injured patients. *Scand J Psychol*. 2000;41:113-121.

334. Scheinberg LC. Multiple sclerosis: therapeutic strategies. *Ann Neurol*. 1994;36(suppl):S122.

335. Schick S, Gahleitner A, Wober-Bingol C, et al. Virchow-Robin spaces in childhood migraine. *Neuroradiology*. 1999;41:283-287.

336. Schnider P, Trattnig S, Kollegger H, Auff E. MR of cerebral Whipple disease. *Am J Neuroradiol*. 1995;16:1328-1329.

337. Schulder M, Sernas T, Mahalick D, Adler R, Cook S. Thalamic stimulation in patients with multiple sclerosis. *Stereotact Funct Neurosurg*. 1999;72:196-201.

338. Schultheis MT, Garay E, De Luca J. The influence of cognitive impairment on driving performance in multiple sclerosis. *Neurology*. 2001;56:1089-1094.

339. Schuurman PR, Bosch DA, Bossuyt PM, et al. A comparison of continuous thalamic stimulation and thalamotomy for suppression of severe tremor. *N Engl J Med*. 2000;342:461-468.

340. Schwankhaus JD, Katz DA, Eldridge R, Schlesinger S, McFarland H. Clinical and pathological features of an autosomal dominant, adult-onset leukodystrophy simulating chronic progressive multiple sclerosis. *Arch Neurol*. 1994;51:757-766.

341. Schwarz S, Mohr A, Knauth M, Wildemann B, Storch-Hagenlocher B. Acute disseminated encephalomyelitis: a follow-up study of 40 adult patients. *Neurology*. 2001;56:1313-1318.

342. Schwid SR, Bever CT. The cost of delaying treatment in multiple sclerosis: what is lost is not regained. *Neurology*. 2001;56:1620.

343. Scott TF, Schramke CJ, Novero J, Chieffe C. Short-term prognosis in early relapsing-remitting multiple sclerosis. *Neurology*. 2000;55:689-693.

344. Shapiro RT. *Symptom Management in Multiple Sclerosis*. New York, NY: Demos Medical Publishing; 1998.

345. Shapiro RT, Schneider DM. Fatigue. In: van den Noort S, Holland NJ, eds. *Multiple Sclerosis in Clinical Practice*. New York, NY: Demos Medical Publishing; 1999:35-40.

346. Sharpe M, Carson A. "Unexplained" somatic symptoms, functional syndromes, and somatization: do we need a paradigm shift? *Ann Intern Med*. 2001;134:926-930.

347. Sibley WA, Bamford CR, Clark K. Clinical viral infections and multiple sclerosis. *Lancet*. 1985;1:1313-1315.

348. Sibley WA, Bamford CR, Clark K, Smith MS, Laguna JF. A prospective study of physical trauma and multiple sclerosis. *J Neurol Neurosurg Psychiatry*. 1991;54:584-589.

349. Silber MH. Sleep disorders. *Neurol Clin*. 2001;19:173-186.

350. Simon JH. Magnetic resonance imaging in the diagnosis of multiple sclerosis, elucidation of disease course, and determining prognosis. In: Burks JS, Johnson KP, eds. *Multiple Sclerosis: Diagnosis, Medical Management, and Rehabilitation*. New York, NY: Demos Medical Publishing; 2000:99-126.

351. Sindern E, Patzold T, Vorgerd M, et al. Adult polyglucosan antibody disease. Case report with predominant involvement of the central and peripheral nervous system and branching enzyme defect in leukocytes (German). *Nervenarzt*. 1999;70:745-749.

352. Smeltzer SC, Skurnick JH, Troiano R, Cook SD, Duran W, Lavietes MH. Respiratory function in multiple sclerosis. Utility of clinical assessment of respiratory muscle function. *Chest*. 1992;101:479-484.

353. Smith JW. Urinary tract infections. In: Hurst JW, ed. *Medicine for the Practicing Physician*. Stamford, Conn: McGraw-Hill Professional Publishing; 1996:354-356.

354. Smith ME, Stone LA, Albert PS, et al. Clinical worsening in multiple sclerosis is associated with increased frequency and area of gadopentetate dimeglumine-enhancing magnetic resonance imaging lesions. *Ann Neurol*. 1993;33:480-490.

355. Smoller JW, Pollack MH, Otto MW, Rosenbaum JF, Kradin RL. Panic anxiety, dyspnea, and respiratory disease. Theoretical and clinical considerations. *Am J Respir Crit Care Med*. 1996;154:6-17.

10

356. Sobel RA. The pathology of multiple sclerosis. *Neurol Clin*. 1995;13:1-21.

357. Soderstrom M, Ya-Ping J, Hillert J, Link H. Optic neuritis: prognosis for multiple sclerosis from MRI, CSF, and HLA findings. *Neurology*. 1998;50:708-714.

358. Sorensen PM. Dysarthria. In: Burks JS, Johnson KP, eds. *Multiple Sclerosis: Diagnosis, Medical Management, and Rehabilitation*. New York, NY: Demos Medical Publishing; 2000:385-404.

359. Spengos K, Schwartz A, Hennerici M. Multifocal cerebral demyelination after magic mushroom abuse. *J Neurol*. 2000;247:224-225.

360. Sriram S, Rodriguez M. Indictment of the microglia as the villain in multiple sclerosis. *Neurology*. 1997;48:464-470.

361. Stanbury RM, Wallace GR, Graham EM. Intermediate uveitis: pars planitis, multiple sclerosis, and retinal vasculitis. *Ophthal Clin North Am*. 1998;11:627-639.

362. Steere AC. Lyme disease. *N Engl J Med*. 2001;345:115-125.

363. Stevens JM, Serva WA, Kendall BE, Valentine AR, Ponsford JR. Chiari malformation in adults: relation of morphological aspects to clinical features and operative outcome. *J Neurol Neurosurg Psychiatry*. 1993;56:1072-1077.

364. Stockhammer G, Felber SR, Zelger B, et al. Sneddon's syndrome: diagnosis by skin biopsy and MRI in 17 patients. *Stroke*. 1993;24:685-690.

365. Stuart WH. Treatment of paroxysmal symptoms. In: Rudick RA, Goodkin DE, eds. *Multiple Sclerosis Therapeutics*. London: Blackwell Science Inc; 1999:547-552.

366. Subbiah P, Wijdicks E, Muenter M, Carter J, Connolly S. Skin lesion with a fatal neurologic outcome (Degos' disease). *Neurology*. 1996;46:636-640.

367. Subramony SH, Filla A. Autosomal dominant spinocerebellar ataxias ad infinitum? *Neurology*. 2001;56:287-289.

368. Surtees R, Leonard J, Austin S. Association of demyelination with deficiency of cerebrospinal-fluid S-adenosylmethionine in inborn errors of methyl-transfer pathway. *Lancet*. 1991;338:1550-1554.

369. Tacconi L, Miles JB. Bilateral trigeminal neuralgia: a therapeutic dilemma. *Br J Neurosurg*. 2000;14:33-39.

370. Tan IL, van Schijndel RA, Pouwels PJ, et al. MR venography of multiple sclerosis. *Am J Neuroradiol*. 2000;21:1039-1042.

371. Tanyel MC, Mancano LD. Neurologic findings in vitamin E deficiency. *Am Fam Physician*. 1997;55:197-201.

372. Templ JI, Ferrer JM, Sevilla MT, Lago A, Mayordomo F, Vilchez JJ. Neurologic complications associated with hepatitis C virus infection. *Neurology*. 1999;53:861-864.

373. Teva Pharmaceutical Industries, press release, September 17,2001.

374. Thadani H, Deacon A, Peters T. Diagnosis and management of porphyria. *BMJ*. 2000;320:1647-1651.

375. Thomas PK, Walker RW, Rudge P, et al. Chronic demyelinating peripheral neuropathy associated with multifocal central nervous system demyelination. *Brain*. 1987;110:53-76.

376. Thorpe JW, Kidd D, Moseley IF, et al. Spinal MRI in patients with suspected multiple sclerosis and negative brain MRI. *Brain*. 1996;119:709-714.

377. Thuomas KA, Moller C, Odkvist LM, Flodin U, Dige N. MR imaging in solvent-induced chronic toxic encephalopathy. *Acta Radiol.* 1996;37:177-179.

378. Tintore M, Rovira A, Martinez MJ, et al. Isolated demyelinating syndromes: comparison of different MR imaging criteria to predict conversion to clinically definite multiple sclerosis. *Am J Neuroradiol.* 2000;21:702-706.

379. Tippett DS, Fishman PS, Panitch HS. Relapsing transverse myelitis. *Neurology.* 1991;41:703-706.

380. Tomoda A, Shiraishi S, Hosoya M, Hamada A, Miike T. Combined treatment with interferon-alpha and ribavirin for subacute sclerosing panencephalitis. *Pediatr Neurol.* 2001;24:54-59.

381. Tourbah A, Piette JC, Iba-Zizen MT, Lyon-Caen O, Godeau P, Frances C. The natural course of cerebral lesions in Sneddon syndrome. *Arch Neurol.* 1997;54:53-60.

382. Tramont EC. Treponema pallidum. In: Mandell GL, Bennett JE, Dolin R, eds. *Principles and Practice of Infectious Diseases.* New York, NY: Churchill Livingstone;2000:2474-2490.

383. Trapp BD, Peterson J, Ransohoff RM, Rudick R, Mork S, Bo L. Axonal transection in the lesions of multiple sclerosis. *N Engl J Med.* 1998;338:278-285.

384. Triantafillidis JK, Kottaras G, Sgourous S, et al. A-beta-lipoproteinemia: clinical and laboratory features, therapeutic manipulations, and follow-up study of three members of a Greek family. *J Clin Gastroenterol.* 1998;26:207-211.

385. Triulzi F, Scotti G. Differential diagnosis of multiple sclerosis: contribution of magnetic resonance techniques. *J Neurol Neurosurg Psychiatry.* 1998;64(suppl 1):S6-S14.

386. Usuki F, Maruyama K. Ataxia caused by mutations in the alpha-tocopherol transfer protein gene. *J Neurol Neurosurg Psychiatry.* 2000;69:254-256.

387. Uziel G, Moroni I, Lamantea E, et al. Mitochondrial disease associated with the T8993G mutation of the mitochondrial ATPase 6 gene: a clinical, biochemical, and molecular study in six families. *J Neurol Neurosurg Psychiatry.* 1997;63:16-22.

388. Van der Knaap MS, Valk J. *Magnetic Resonance of Myelin, Myelination, and Myelin Disorders* (Second Edition). Berlin: Springer Verlag; 1995.

389. Van Walderveen MAA, Barkhof F. Measures of T1 and T2 relaxation. In: Rudick RA, Goodkin DE, eds. *Multiple Sclerosis Therapeutics.* London: Blackwell Science Inc; 1999:91-106.

390. von Herbay A, Ditton HJ, Schuhmacher F, Maiwald M. Whipple's disease: staging and monitoring by cytology and polymerase chain reaction analysis of cerebrospinal fluid. *Gastroenterology.* 1997;113:434-441.

391. Wang FI, Hinton DR, Gilmore W, Trousdale MD, Fleming JO. Sequential infection of glial cells by the murine hepatitis virus JHM strain (MHV-4) leads to a characteristic distribution of demyelination. *Lab Invest.* 1992;66:744-754.

392. Waxman SG. Pathophysiology of multiple sclerosis. In: Cook SD, ed. *Handbook of Multiple Sclerosis (Neurological Disease and Therapy, Vol 8).* New York, NY: Marcel Dekker; 1990:219-249.

393. Waxman SG. Peripheral nerve abnormalities in multiple sclerosis. *Muscle Nerve.* 1993;16:1-5.

10

394. Weber F, Conrad B. Chronic encephalitis and Eales disease. *J Neurology.* 1993;240:299-301.

395. Wechsler B, Dell'Isola B, Vidailhet M, et al. MRI in 31 patients with Behcet's disease and neurological involvement: prospective study with clinical correlation. *J Neurol Neurosurg Psychiatry.* 1993;56: 793-798.

396. Weight DG, Bigler ED. Neuroimaging in psychiatry. *Psychiatr Clin North Am.* 1998;21:725-759.

397. Weihl CC, Roos RP. Creutzfeldt-Jakob disease, new variant creutzfeldt-jakob disease, and bovine spongiform encephalopathy. *Neurol Clin.* 1999;17:835-859.

398. Weil S, Reifenberger G, Dudel C, Yousry TA, Schriever S, Noachtar S. Cerebroretinal vasculopathy mimicking a brain tumor: a case of a rare hereditary syndrome. *Neurology.* 1999;53:629-631.

399. Weinshenker BG. Therapeutic plasma exchange. In: Rudick RA, Goodkin DE, eds. *Multiple Sclerosis Therapeutics.* London: Blackwell Science Inc; 1999:323-333.

400. Weinshenker BG, O'Brien PC, Petterson TM, et al. A randomized trial of plasma exchange in acute central nervous system inflammatory demyelinating disease. *Ann Neurol.* 1999;46:878-886.

401. Weinshenker BG. Progressive forms of MS: classification streamlined or consensus overturned? *Lancet* 2000;355:162-163.

402. Weinshenker BG, Lucchinetti CF. Acute leukoencephalopathies. *Neurologist.* 1998;4:148-166.

403. Wenzel KC. Ad-vocational issues. In: Burks JS, Johnson KP, eds. *Multiple Sclerosis: Diagnosis, Medical Management, and Rehabilitation.* New York, NY: Demos Medical Publishing;2000:555-561.

404. Whooley MA, Simon GE. Managing depression in medical outpatients. *N Engl J Med.* 2000;343:1942-1950.

405. Wilke WS. Can fibromyalgia and chronic fatigue syndrome be cured by surgery? *Cleve Clin J Med.* 2001;68:277-279.

406. Williams GJ, Witt PL. Comparative study of the pharmacodynamic and pharmacologic effects of Betaseron and AVONEX. *J Interferon Cytokine Res.* 1998;18:967-975.

407. Williamson RA, Burgoon MP, Owens GP, et al. Anti-DNA antibodies are a major component of the intrathecal B cell response in multiple sclerosis. *Proc Natl Acad Sci U S A.* 2001;98:1793-1798.

408. Wingerchuk DM, Hogancamp WF, O'Brien PC, Weinshenker BG. The clinical course of neuromyelitis optica (Devic's syndrome). *Neurology.* 1999;53:1107-1114.

409. Wingerchuk DM, Lucchinetti CF, Noseworthy JH. Multiple sclerosis: current pathophysiological concepts. *Lab Invest.* 2001;81:263-281.

410. Yaqub BA, al-Deeb SM, Daif AK, et al. Bickerstaff brainstem encephalitis. A grave non-demyelinating disease with benign prognosis. *J Neurol Sci.* 1990;96:29-40.

411. Young C. Symptomatic management: Ataxia, tremor and fatigue. In: Hawkins C, Wolinsky JS, eds. *Principles of Treatments in Multiple Sclerosis.* Oxford: Butterworth –Heinemann Medical; 2000:228-257.

412. Young EJ. Brucella species. In: Mandell GL, Bennett JE, Dolin R, eds. *Mandell, Douglas, and Bennett's Principles and Practice of Infectious Diseases (2 Volume Set).* New York, NY: Churchill Livingstone; 2000:2386-2393.

413. Young RR. Spastic paresis. In: Burks JS, Johnson KP, eds. *Multiple Sclerosis: Diagnosis, Medical Management, and Rehabilitation*. New York, NY: Demos Medical Publishing; 2000:299-306.

414. Young WF, Weaver M, Mishra B. Surgical outcome in patients with coexisting multiple sclerosis and spondylosis. *Acta Neurol Scand*. 1999;100:84-87.

415. Younger DS, Kass RM. Vasculitis and the nervous system. Historical perspective and overview. *Neurol Clin*. 1997;15:737-758.

416. Ziemssen F, Sindern E, Schroder JM, et al. Novel missense mutations in the glycogen-branching enzyme gene in adult polyglucosan body disease. *Ann Neurol*. 2000;47:536-540.

Additional References:

417. Chang A, Tourtellotte WW, Rudick R, Trapp BD. Premyelinating oligodendrocytes in chronic lesions of multiple sclerosis. *N Engl J Med*. 2002;346:165-173.

418. Brex PA, Ciccarelli O, O'Riordan JI, Sailer M, Thompson AJ, Miller DH. A longitudinal study of abnormalities on MRI and disability from multiple sclerosis. *N Engl J Med*. 2002;346:158-164

419. Goodin DS, Frohman EM, Garmany GP, et al. Disease modifying therapies in multiple sclerosis: Report of the Therapeutics and Technology Assessment Subcommittee of the American Academy of Neurology and the MS Council for Clinical Practice Guidelines. *Neurology*. 2002;58:169-178.

10

Note: Page numbers in *italics* indicate figures;
page numbers followed by t refer to tables.

11

11

11

11

11

11

11

11

11

11

11

11

11

11

11

11